MIRED
IN THE
HEALTH CARE
MORASS

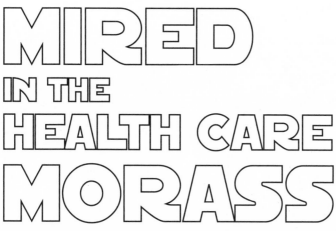

MIRED IN THE HEALTH CARE MORASS

An Alaskan Takes on America's Dysfunctional
Medical System for his Uninsured Daughter

NEIL DAVIS

Ester Republic Press
Alaska-Yukon Press
Ester, Alaska

Mired in the Health Care Morass: An Alaskan Takes on America's Dysfunctional Medical System for his Uninsured Daughter

Cover photo by the author of a permafrost bog near Cantwell, Alaska (image manipulated in Photoshop).

Published by the Ester Republic Press
PO Box 24, Ester AK 99725
visit us on line at www.esterrepublic.com

Printed in the United States of America by Thomson-Shore, Inc.
an employee-owned company

first printing, February 2008: 1,500 copies
second printing, September 2008: 3,000 copies

ISBN 978-0-9749221-4-0 (paperback)
Library of Congress Control Number: 2007943962

member of the Green Press Initiative

MORASS: "often used figuratively of a difficult, troublesome, or perplexing state of affairs."

—WEBSTER'S DICTIONARY

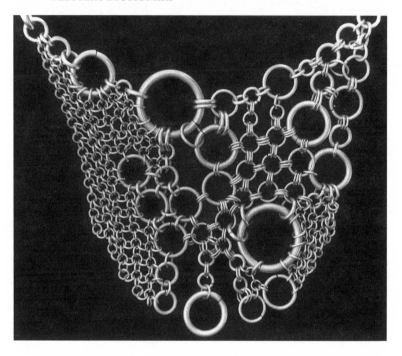

Contents

1

*Nothing can be loved or hated
unless it is first known.*

—LEONARDO DA VINCI

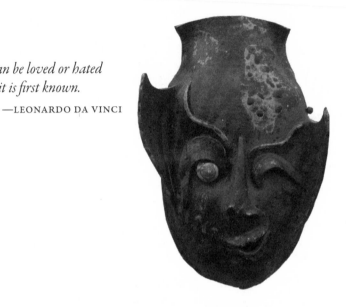

Introduction: The First Warning Bell

My first hint that something was wrong came when I glanced at the medical bill on top of the stack on my desk. One entry showed a charge of $1,224 for a 50-mg injection of carboplatin, a chemotherapy drug, and a few lines farther down was a similar entry but there the price was $1,428. Then I noticed that the first injection had been administered by one doctor, and the second injection by a different one. What the heck is going on here? I thought to myself. Does the price depend on the doctor, and if that is so, what determines the amount the doctor charges? I need to look into this.

And so that afternoon in January 2005 began my education into the mysterious realm of medical costs and billing practices. During the next two years, this educational process would also teach me more than I wanted to know about the American healthcare system. Looking back, I now almost cannot believe how naïve I was at the beginning, but as I went along I began to comprehend that my initial ignorance was shared by many of my friends and, in fact, probably by most Americans. Nearly all of us knew that the American medical system was terribly expensive and getting more expensive by the day. We were hearing that it was a dysfunctional system, but we did not know enough about it to really understand it or how to fix it.

Having now gone through this process of self-education, I can state in very few sentences what I think are the real problems with American health care, and how we can fix the system. So can a number of others who have examined the healthcare system in detail, and for them I would simply be preaching to the choir. Most others probably would not take my statements seriously because they so differ from what is typically seen in the press. So I put that discussion off until later, after readers have a chance to see why I reached these conclusions, ones that they are likely to come to on their own before seeing mine.

As I went along I found highly useful several recently available books on the topics covered here. They include:

Health Care Meltdown: Confronting the myths and fixing the system, by Robert H. LeBow (Chambersburg, Pennsylvania: Alan C. Hood & Company, 2004, ISBN 0-911469-23-0, paper, $15). LeBow, an Idaho physician with broad experience in international health care, died at age 63, just before this book came out. Several years earlier he was in a bicycle accident that rendered him quadriplegic.

The Truth About Drug Companies: How they deceive us and what to do about it, by Marcia Angell (New York: Random House, 2004, ISBN 0-375-50846-5 cloth, $24.95). Dr. Angell is former editor in chief of *The New England Journal of Medicine*.

Falling Through the Safety Net: Americans without health insurance, by John Geyman (Monroe, Maine: Common Courage Press, 2005, ISBN 1-56751-254-2 paper, $18.95). Dr. Geyman is professor emeritus of family medicine at the University of Washington School of Medicine, where he was the department chairman.

The Corporate Transformation of Health Care: Can the public interest still be served? by John Geyman (New York: Springer Publishing Company, 2004, ISBN 0-8261-2466-6 paper, $41.95).

Uninsured in America: Life and death in the land of opportunity, by Susan Starr Sereo and Rushinka Ferdanopulle (Berkeley, University of California Press, ISBN 978-0-520-24442-9 paper, $24.95). Sereo is research director of the Religion, Health and Healing Initiative at the Center for the Study of World Religions, Harvard University, and Fernandopulle is executive director of the Harvard Interfaculty Program for Health Systems.

My book differs from these others in that it is written by a **consumer*** rather than a professional **provider** of medical services, and from a consumer's viewpoint. I have structured the book around the experiences of our family that began when our adult daughter Patricia was diagnosed with lung cancer. Another difference from the other books is that this one delves deeply into many of the financial details of the medical profession, particularly those that affected us directly. Yet another difference is that the setting of this book is Alaska. Alaska's large land area and low population affect the delivery of medical care and make it more costly than in most other parts of the United States. Nevertheless, the experiences we have in this state are those of people everywhere in the country, and so the lessons our family have learned here in the northern outback have broad application elsewhere in America.

I must warn that this book travels a road paved with many prickly details that most of us would prefer to ignore. My experience, however, is that a useful understanding of the whole comes only from looking at those details. A quick sniff at the air does not allow one to savor the true smell—you really need to get down and rub your nose in it. That requires looking at specific information, and that often comes only from looking at numbers. So as you read on, prepare yourself to look at a lot of numbers.

---

* At first appearance in the text, terms such as this are set in bold type to indicate that they appear in the Glossary.

Americans now spend a staggering $200 billion on prescription drugs, and that figure is growing at about 12 percent a year.

—MARCIA ANGELL,
FORMER EDITOR IN CHIEF OF THE
NEW ENGLAND JOURNAL OF MEDICINE

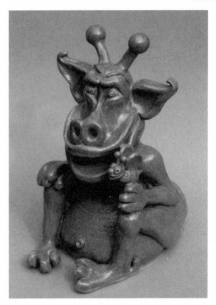

My Introduction to Drugs and Medical Billing

The Opening Salvo

The story really begins in early November 2004 when Patricia, the elder daughter of our three offspring, told us that she had just been diagnosed with Stage III non-small-cell lung cancer.

At that time Patricia was a 52-year-old self-employed artist and part-time teacher who had no heath insurance in effect. She had been covered by health insurance most of her life, by family policies during childhood and during her college years, and later as the wife of a university teacher. A divorce terminated that coverage, and for some years, as she struggled to maintain herself and a son, she had gone without any insurance coverage whatsoever because she thought she could not afford it. Aware that she was following a treacherous path, Patricia had taken a part-time job for a small Alaska airline hoping to get health insurance that would begin after she had been employed full-time for six months. Her work as a filing clerk allowed her to continue on with her artistic endeavors, which were far-ranging but mainly involved metalsmithing, with one-of-a-kind silver jewelry her specialty. (Because this story relates to what happened to Patricia, I include at section headings photographs of her artwork, and feature a group of clay figures she created during the first six months of 2006. She was then undergoing chemotherapy, so she called them her Chemo-brain series.)

Three months into her new job, Patricia was experiencing symptoms that should have sent her to the doctor, but she chose to wait until her health insurance would become effective. Then the symptoms became worse, and she finally did go and learned that there was a tumor in her lung. The medics sprang into action immediately. One team operated only to discover that the cancerous tumor was too close to her aorta to be removed surgically, and so chemotherapy and radiation treatments commenced. By the end of December 2005, two **hospital**s and nine different doctors and laboratories had been involved in her care.

It was at this point that I entered the picture, with the idea of paying Patricia's medical bills, at least to the extent our finances permitted. I thought she had enough on her mind without the worry of having to pay bills, which by then amounted to many tens of thousands of dollars. Patricia had tried: she gave one doctor $300, all she could afford just then. "Give me the bills," I told her. "I will take care of them from now on."

If I'm going to pay these bills I'd best take a look at them, I told myself. So I sat down at my desk with a stack of them before me, and realized that there was something very odd about that bill at the top of the pile.

Having no background in medicine, and having never before given more than cursory examination to my own medical bills, I found the task daunting. I was confused by a lot of new terminology and, right away, an apparent contradiction. That first bill listed the charge for a 50-milligram (mg) injection of carboplatin as $1,224 in one place and $1,428 in another. I didn't even know what carboplatin was, and so it seemed to be a good idea to find that out, and also to find out what carboplatin really costs on the open market.

Searching the Internet, I soon learned that carboplatin and two other drugs, Taxol and Anzemet, were a combination often used to treat cancer **patient**s. And, yes, there on Patricia's bills were charges for those other two drugs as well. Patricia was receiving other medications also, but these three were the most expensive, so I decided to ignore the others and concentrate my efforts on carboplatin, Taxol, and Anzemet.

My initial finding was stunning. On the world market I could buy 50 mg of carboplatin in bulk (2,000 doses) for $13.50 per dose. This drug obviously did not cost much to manufacture, and I found that a major pharmacy retailer in New York was selling it in small quantities for $61.36 per dose. Yet Patricia was being charged, in one case, $1,224, and in another $1,428? Clearly, something was radically wrong here.

Armed with what I had learned about the pricing of carboplatin and the two related expensive drugs Anzemet and Taxol, I visited Patricia's oncologist to ask why he and his associates were billing her so much for these drugs.

He wasn't really charging that much, he explained, it was just that the billings Patricia had been receiving didn't tell the full story. It was akin to a Y2K problem: his office used a computer to generate the billings, and there was not enough room on the billing forms to tell how many dosage units were involved. The billings of $1,224 for carboplatin in one case and for $1,428 in the other were because six dosage units were given in the one case and seven in the other. The charge was really only $204 per dosage unit.

So here was one little lesson in medical billing practice: the biller often feels no obligation to provide all the information that an uninsured patient might want. In this case, the doctor's billing personnel saw no need to change their billing form over to one that would provide full information. Evidently they thought the patient should just pay the bill—never mind the details.

But even at $204 per 50-mg unit of carboplatin, the charge seemed to be too high, I suggested, and also for Taxol and Anzemet. The doctor was a bit vague, but he gave me the impression that many uninsured patients could not pay for the drugs they received, and so the high charges to Patricia were to help compensate. I could understand that, but then I was wondering why Patricia, now too sick to work enough to pay for her own upkeep, was being asked to help pay for the medical treatment of other patients. The doctor then offered an out: He would charge nothing for the drugs if I would replace them, and he would write a set of prescriptions to make that possible. Cooperating even more, the doctor arranged for his billing personnel to give me copies of the full billings like those that go to **Medicare**, **Medicaid**, and private insurance companies when a patient has such coverage. These bills gave all the details, including the coding information on each drug and medical procedure performed.

My Big Drug Purchase

Armed with the prescriptions, I checked prices at several local pharmacies, and then homed in on a source named RxUSA, a federally registered pharmacy supplier in New York state. I saw that I could perhaps save a little money by buying from a Canadian source, but I did not want there to be any question whatsoever about the quality or other aspects of the replacement drugs I would be buying. (Actually, the recently enacted Medicare Prescription Drug Improvement and Modernization Act of 2003 made it illegal for me to buy prescription drugs outside the country, but I did not know that.)

I ordered the drugs to replace those injected during the first eight weeks' round of treatments, and then a second batch to be injected in the next round of four treatments, this time with much higher dosages. The injections during the first round were carboplatin, 300 mg; Taxol, 90 mg; Anzemet, 100 mg. The next four treatments would be carboplatin, 1,200 mg; Taxol, 400 mg; Anzemet, 100 mg. (That first round of treatments had been tough on Patricia, and the next round was going to be even more difficult for her, but happily, it would produce positive effects.) The following two tables show the overall result of the drug purchase. Table 2.1, included here mainly for the benefit of professionals used to dealing with dosage units, gives cost information in those terms. Table 2.2 gives summary information for the first two rounds of Patricia's chemotherapy treatments.

My early researches also revealed how much Medicare would have allowed to be paid for the injections had Patricia been old enough or so situated that she had Medicare coverage. The **Medicare allowance** information is included in the tables.

Table 2.2 shows that over the course of the first two rounds of treatments given during late 2004 and early 2005, Patricia received billings for $50,701. Assuming the Medicare 2004 allowances, were Patricia covered by Medicare, the maximum payment to the prescribing physician would have been $31,722 or, if the 2005 rates were to pertain, the physician would have

Table 2.1 - Carboplatin, Taxol, and Anzemet injections, showing charges and costs per billing dosage unit and Medicare Allowance Limits.

Drug Injected	Billing Dosage Unit	Billed to Patricia Per Unit	What I Paid Per Unit	Medicare Allowance 2004	Medicare Allowance 2005
Carboplatin Code J9045	50 mg	$204.00	$61.36	$125.47*	
Taxol, (Onxol, Paclitaxil) Code J9265	30 mg	$255.90	$25.73	$138.28	$25.84
Anzemet (Dolasetron) Code J1260	10 mg	$23.00	$9.16	$14.24	$16.45
Overall Totals		$482.90	$96.25	$278.00	$167.76

*Assumed to be same both years.

Table 2.2 - Carboplatin, Taxol, and Anzemet injections, two rounds of treatment for Patricia.

Drug Injected	Total Dosage	Billed to Patricia	Total I Paid for the Drugs	Medicare Allowance 2004	Medicare Allowance 2005
Carboplatin	6900 mg	$28,152	$13,014	$17,315	$17,315
Taxol, (Onxol, Paclitaxil)	2320 mg	$19,789	$2,130	$10,694	$1,998
Anzemet (Dolasetron)	1200 mg	$2,760	$533	$1,709	$1,974
Overall Totals		$50,701	$15,677	$31,722	$23,292

received $23,292. The table also shows that I was able to buy the drugs in the United States for far less than either figure, $15,677. Assuming that the physician could buy the drugs at the same price I paid, his allowed markup for his Medicare patients was substantial in both 2004 ($16,045) and 2005 ($7,625). The big difference between the Medicare allowances in the two years is due to the radical reduction in 2005 of the previous unreasonably high Medicare allowance for the drug Taxol. (The allowance was lowered when it was realized that the drug's marketer, Bristol-Myers Squibb, had been gouging Medicare and the public by vastly overpricing the drug, one actually developed by the government and then licensed to Bristol-Myers Squibb.)

Having just saved ($50,701 - $15,677 =) $35,024 by my first venture into the prescription drug business, I should have felt pretty good about it. However, along the way I had done some reading about the pharmaceutical industry that was more than a little unsettling.

Tidbits about Carboplatin, Taxol, Anzemet, and Drugs in General

Here are a couple of quotations from some articles I read, mostly on the Internet:

"Bristol-Myers Squibb's Taxol sales are expected to be about $1 billion this year [1997], making the drug an enormous profit center for the company....The cost of [ready-to-sell] Taxol is $0.40/mg. Bristol-Myers Squibb sells it wholesale for $4.87/mg....Bristol-Myers Squibb is lobbying the United States government to take trade sanctions against South Africa, Canada, Australia, Argentina, the Netherlands and other countries which have approved **generic** versions of Taxol, the NIH developed cancer drug currently sold by Bristol-Myers Squibb." [1]

"For years, federal investigators have been churning out reports showing that physicians are overcharging Medicare for chemotherapy drugs used to treat cancer patients. Doctors who pay only $7.75 for a single dose of Vincasar, for example, are reimbursed at a rate of $700 under Medicare. The government covers $560, and the Medicare patient pays $140." [2]

The second article goes on to say that President Clinton tried to trim the Medicare overpayments, which are estimated to cost American taxpayers $2 billion a year, but intense pressure from drug manufacturers and oncologists led legislators in 1997 to thumb their noses at Clinton by tying the reimbursements to the **"average wholesale price." [AWP]**.

> Despite its name, AWP is not the average price paid by wholesale purchasers. Instead it serves as a kind of 'sticker price' used by the drug companies to open price negotiations, and it far exceeds what doctors actually pay for the drugs.

> The drug manufacturers soon discovered that they could sell more of their drugs by simply inflating the AWP figure. The higher these companies set AWP, the bigger the profit they could offer doctors and hospitals who used their products to treat Medicare patients.

> For **outpatient** drugs, some members of Congress say Medicare should follow the example of the **Veterans Administration**, which awards contracts to the wholesaler that offers to sell a drug to the VA for the lowest price...For half of [24 studied] drugs...Medicare pays more than double the VA price...

> Medicare pays about $173.49 for 30 milligrams of Taxol... while the VA pays only $107.59.

That was before 2005, when I paid just $27.54 for 30 mg of the generic version of Taxol (paclitaxil) purchased from the New York pharmacy supplier RxUSA. In 1998, Medicare was paying $84.16 for a 50-mg dose of carboplatin, and the Veterans Administration was paying $39.50.[3] In 2005, I paid $61.36.

As I dug into what might be determining the price of prescription drugs, I learned that these tidbits were just little chips off the tip of the pharmaceutical industry iceberg sticking up through the murky waters of the American healthcare system.

---

1. James P. Love, Testimony before the U.S. Senate, October 1997; www.cptech. org/pharm/senhregd.html.

2. *St. Petersburg Times* (Florida), July 14, 2002.

3. Department of Health and Human Services, Office of Inspector General, document OEI-03-97-00293, November 1998.

3

*O, it is excellent
To have a giant's strength;
but it is tyrannous
To use it like a giant.*

—WILLIAM SHAKESPEARE

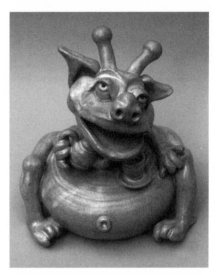

The Powerful Pharmaceutical Industry

Financial Aspects of the Industry

I found that a major source of information about the giant pharmaceutical industry is the recent book, *The Truth About the Drug Companies: How they deceive us and what to do about it*,[4] by Marcia Angell, former editor in chief of *The New England Journal of Medicine* and now a member of Harvard Medical School's Department of Social Medicine. Much of the information presented in this chapter comes from that book.

Worldwide, the pharmaceutical industry is a financial giant with $400 billion in sales, and the American consumption of prescription drugs accounts for half of that. It is the most profitable of all industries in the United States, with profits equaling 25 percent of sales.

In 2001, the ten American drug companies in the Fortune 500 had the highest net return: 18.5 percent of sales, 16.3 percent of assets, and 33.2 percent of equity, whereas the median net income of all **Fortune 500** companies was only 3.3 percent. In 2002, the combined profit for these ten companies ($35.9 billion) was more than that of all other 490 Fortune 500 companies together, $33.7 billion. The five European pharmaceutical giants—GlaxoSmithKline, AstraZeneca, Novartis, Roche, and Aventis—had similar profits.

Chief executive officer earnings in the pharmaceutical industry are large. In 2001, the Bristol-Myers Squibb CEO received $75 million in salary and $76 million in stock options, while the Wyeth chairman received a salary of $40 million and $40 million in stock options.

From 1980 to 2000 drug sales in the United States tripled.

In 2001, the drug companies had the largest lobby in Washington. Its 675 members outnumbered the members of Congress. In 2002, 26 of these lobbyists were former members of Congress, and 342 had been congressional staffers or otherwise connected with government officials.

Big Pharma Companies: Primarily Marketing Machines

In 2000, drug company expenditures for marketing and administration amounted to 36 percent of sales income, but, again according to Dr. Angell, only 14 percent went for **research and development (R&D)**. Thus the expenditure for marketing and administration was two and one-half times that for research and development. The companies evidently think they do not need to invest much in R&D; instead they depend heavily upon government, universities, and small biotech firms for innovation. At least a third of their drugs come from universities and small biotech firms.

Much of the innovation and early-phase work of bringing a drug to market—the research part of R&D—is funded by the **National Institutes of Health (NIH)** or other government-sponsored organizations.

Of seventy-eight drugs approved by the **Food and Drug Administration (FDA)** in 2002, only seventeen contained new active ingredients, and only seven were classified by FDA as improvements over older drugs. Not one of these came from a major drug company.

The drug companies claim that it costs them $800 million to bring a new drug to market, but Angell says this is a major exaggeration. For the reasons given above, she suggests the true cost to them is less than $100 million.

In short, Big Pharma is not telling the public the truth when it claims that the high price of the pharmaceuticals it sells are due to R&D costs. High profits and large marketing costs are the true reason the public has to pay such high prices for pharmaceuticals.

Bringing a Drug to Market

As the phrase "Research and Development" implies, bringing a drug to market involves two phases: the research phase, and the development phase.

The *research phase* involves two steps: The first entails learning about a disease or condition that might be treated with a drug. This part of the process is almost all done by universities and government laboratories and is government funded. The second step is to discover or synthesize a potentially useful molecule or biotech product for treating the disease or condition. This work takes place in universities, government laboratories, small biotech firms, and in laboratories operated by the major pharmaceutical companies.

The *development phase* begins upon completion of the research phase, and at this stage the pharmaceutical companies that will sell the drugs begin to play a greater role in the overall process. The development phase also involves two steps: the preclinical stage and the clinical stage.

Preclinical stage—The first part of the development phase, the preclinical stage, involves the search for promising drug candidates and study of their properties by testing in animals and cell cultures. Only about one in a thousand candidates survive this stage. Normally, patenting of the survivors is now undertaken, and that gives 25 years of protection for the owner of the resulting patents. To provide as many years of protection as possible after marketing begins, it behooves the patent owners to move through the subsequent clinical stage as rapidly as possible.

The *clinical stage* entails testing on humans, and it has four phases:

▶ **Phase I**—Give the new drug to a small number of persons, usually volunteers, to determine dosages and safety.

▶ **Phase II**—Test on a few hundred patients with the relevant disease.

▶ **Phase III**—Test on a large number of patients (hundreds to thousands) to evaluate the drug's safety and effectiveness using comparison groups of patients. Assuming the drug passes the test, at the end of this stage the drug goes to market.

▶ **Phase IV**—Post-marketing studies to find new uses for old drugs to expand the market and perhaps extend patents. Twenty-five percent of all clinical trials are Phase IV. One current example is Pfizer's Phase IV testing of the infamous and highly profitable drug Viagra (sildenafil citrate) for treating children with cardiovascular problems.

At any one time approximately 80,000 clinical trials are underway. The drug companies usually contract with private companies called **Contract Research Organizations** to establish networks of physicians who are paid to administer the drugs and collect the required information. Worldwide, approximately 1,000 Contract Research Organizations are in operation, and they do a $7 billion business annually. The involved physicians make money as well: most of the tested patients receive some money, but the doctors do much better, receiving an average of $7,000 per patient. Angell [5] cites one trial in which participating physicians were paid $12,000 for each enrolled patient, plus another $30,000 for the sixth patient enrolled.

In the United States, the Food and Drug Administration's involvement with drugs begins at the clinical stage. Drug companies must file an application to begin testing, and upon completion of a trial, file an application for approval. The FDA does not require that a drug work better than one already approved for a particular disease or condition, only that it work better than a placebo. A drug might undergo several clinical trials that do not demonstrate that the drug is better than a placebo, yet receive FDA approval *if one or two other trials do!* Marketers of **generic drugs** do not have to perform clinical trials to prove safety and effectiveness because it is assumed that the marketers of the branded drugs have already accomplished that.[6]

Tricks of the Trade for Extending Patents

Angell notes that the lifeblood of the major pharmaceutical companies is the monopoly that the government confers to them in the form of patents, and that competition from generic drugs comes into play only after patents expire. Therefore the companies do everything possible to extend their patents.

One technique they use is to obtain multiple patents on a drug, easily done because they can obtain patents on various features of a drug such as: 1) its chemical composition; 2) the method of use of the drug for a particular condition such as heart failure or depression; 3) the formulation of the drug; i.e., its form as a liquid or capsule, or its method of application: orally, topically, or by injection; and 4) the process of manufacturing the drug. It is even possible to patent the color of coating on a pill or capsule. So the companies typically take out multiple patents on a drug so as to be able to sue a generic manufacturer for allegedly infringing on any one of the patents. Such a suit puts an automatic 30-month hold on the sale of the generic. Another ploy for extending patents is to test a drug for some use other than the one granted in the original patent—for example, using a drug on children that has been approved only for adults, or using it to treat a disease or condition different from that for which the drug was originally approved.

Yet another approach is for a company to petition to sell a prescription drug over the counter because this adds an extra three-year exclusivity for the drug.

Marketing Tricks

Big Pharma has an extensive bag of tricks for increasing the sales of prescription drugs.

- ► *Direct advertising to consumers*— From reading magazines and watching television, everybody is familiar with, if not sick of, this ploy. Much money is spent on such advertising.
- ► *Providing free samples*—By giving out $11 billion worth of free samples each year, the industry hopes to hook customers on certain drugs.
- ► *Using sales representatives*—In 2001, the industry had 88,000 reps traveling around the country to visit doctors and hawk drugs to them by means of gifts and discounts on drugs. The number amounts to one rep for every five or six doctors.[7] The industry also pays the doctors several hundred dollars each day to let the reps follow them around as they see patients. When you see an attractive, sharply dressed young man or woman visiting your doctor's office, or following him on his rounds, likely you have just seen a drug rep.
- ► *Employing prescription-tracking companies*—Buying information from pharmacies on doctors' prescription profiles target them better for the drug reps.
- ► *Hiring Medical Education and Communication Companies (MECCs)*—For the purpose of inducing doctors to prescribe certain drugs, pharmaceutical companies hire **Medical Education and Communication Companies (MECCs)**. Some of the approximately 100 for-profit MECCs now in operation are owned by large advertising firms.
- ► *Promoting consumer groups*—Big Pharma fosters or organizes consumer groups with the expectation that they will help "educate" consumers in the use of certain drugs.

- ▶ *Paying doctors to talk up a drug*—The marketing of drugs for "off-label" (unapproved) uses is illegal, but prescription for the off-label uses is not, so to promote those uses the pharmaceutical companies pay doctors to talk the drugs up to other doctors in ways that skirt both antikickback laws and laws against off-label marketing.

- ▶ *Drafting articles for publication*—Drug company personnel draft articles favorable to their products and then pay doctors to publish them.

- ▶ *Sponsoring "medical education"*—In 2001, drug companies used marketing funds to pay for over 60 percent of the ongoing medical education that doctors needed to stay abreast of advances in medicine. The companies hire MECCs to organize educational seminars, prepare teaching material and provide speakers. How unbiased such education might be is a worthy question.

- ▶ *Disease mongering*—Big Pharma routinely campaigns to widen the boundaries of treatable illness inappropriately by inventing new diseases and generating names for common conditions simply for marketing purposes. These cons on the public include Pfizer's erectile dysfunction, acid reflux disease, restless leg syndrome, social anxiety disorder, irritable bowel disorder, generalized anxiety disorder, Eli Lily's premenstrual dysphoric disorder (PMDD), Pfizer's female sexual dysfunction, and Proctor & Gamble's hypoactive sexual desire disorder.*

---

* That's hypo, not hyper—meaning too little, not too much sexual desire, the latter a condition supposedly affecting the crews of long-at-sea whaling ships back in the 1800s, and purportedly treated by adding saltpeter to their food. If the drug companies thought that the afflicted persons would buy drugs to alleviate the condition, no doubt they would have by now also invented hyperactive sexual disorder. Or as I think about it more, it occurs to me that perhaps they could sell some patentable form of saltpeter to those persons the ads say should consult their physicians if they maintain erections for more than four hours after taking Viagra and similar drugs—antidotal downers, so to speak.

Direct consumer advertising is so effective that the top thirteen pharmaceutical companies spent a total of $13.8 billion just on this effort in 2004 and again in 2005. That is less, but not much less, than the $16 billion in the nation's space program annual budget, so this is indeed a massive effort. In 2005, the top spenders were Johnson & Johnson ($2.2 billion), GlaxoSmithKline ($2.2 billion), Pfizer ($2.1 billion), and Novartis ($1.2 billion).[8]

The prescription and over-the-counter drug business is particularly profitable in the United States where, unlike in other countries, drug prices and profits are not regulated. In countries where prices are regulated, the drug cost to consumers is typically half that in the United States. Big Pharma's high profitability depends in large part on this unregulated market, so the industry wants no changes. Fearing that Americans might at some point recognize that the cost of pharmaceuticals is a major contributor to the unreasonably high cost of the American healthcare system, the industry does all it can to dissuade them from reaching that conclusion and acting upon it. Through its trade organization PhRMA (Pharmaceutical Research & Manufacturers of America), the industry maintains an ongoing lobby and propaganda effort. PhRMA's $164-million budget for 2004 makes for interesting reading:[9]

- ▸ $72.7 million for lobbying on Capitol Hill (helping to maintain the 635 industry lobbyists there),
- ▸ $48.7 million for lobbying at the state level,
- ▸ $17.5 million for fighting price controls and protecting patents in foreign countries,
- ▸ $15.8 million for fighting "a union-driven initiative in Ohio which would lower drug prices for uninsured persons,"
- ▸ $4.9 million to lobby the Food & Drug Administration,
- ▸ $2.0 million to pay research and policy organizations "to build intellectual capital and generate a higher volume of messages from credible sources" sympathetic to the industry,

► $1.0 million to fund a standing network of economists to speak against US drug price controls,

► $1.0 million to "change the Canadian health care system." [It's too regulated and therefore not profitable enough to suit Big Pharma's tastes.]

The Bottom Line for Big Pharma

Attesting to the success of the pharmaceutical industry's lobbying and propaganda efforts is the passage of the 2,065-page Medicare Prescription Drug Improvement and Modernization Act of 2003, Public Law 108-173, occasionally referred to as "the no lobbyist left behind act." The act is lucrative for the pharmaceutical and insurance industries because it guarantees them payment through **Medicare D** for substantial portions of their billings to the public, and it prevents Medicare from negotiating drug prices in the same fashion as the Veterans Administration, which is able to negotiate prices downward to about half of what Medicare pays. It also prevents Americans from skirting the high prices by making it illegal for them to buy drugs in Canada or elsewhere. In April 2007, the PhRMA organization was conducting a major advertising and lobbying effort to keep Congress from eliminating this lucrative provision of the act. Even here in Alaska, the outback of America, PhRMA placed full-page ads in the newspapers to convince us not to let Congress screw around with the lucrative (for them) provisions of the Medicare Prescription Drug Improvement and Modernization Act of 2003.

As noted a few pages back, despite its claims that the high cost of drugs is due to the cost of research and development, the industry's actual R&D cost is far less than half its advertising and administrative costs. Dr. Marcia Angell suggests that the relatively small drug company expenditure for R&D and the way that money is spent may spell doom for future high profits. Instead of investing more of its too-small R&D effort in developing innovative new drugs, the industry is placing much effort in bringing to market so-called **"me-too" drugs**. These are merely minor variants of existing drugs containing no new active ingredients and which may be no more or even less effective than those already on the market. The only requirement is that they be better than placebos. Dr. Angell noted that two-thirds of all new patented drugs are of this variety. The consequence is that very few new high-profit drugs are coming available, and so the industry's high profits might well plummet. You can bet that PhRMA and its member companies will do their best not to let that happen.[†]

† Today it is common practice for reporters and commentators in the media to disclose any holdings or connections they or their employers have in industries and organizations they are discussing. Following suit, I admit here that since I began learning about the profitability of the pharmaceutical industry I have been investing in that area—and, oh boy, has it paid off!

4. Angell, Marcia, *The Truth About the Drug Companies: How they deceive us and what to do about it* (New York, Random House, 2004).
5. Angell, 2004, loc. cit., p. 31.
6. Angell, Ibid., p. 32.
7. Angell, Marcia, Don't be deceived by drug company tactics, *BOTTOM LINE Health*, March 2005, p. 11.
8. Imedia Connection, How Pharma reaches its audience; www.imediaconnection.com/content/10832.asp.
9. Harvey, Ken, *Australian Review of Public Affairs*, March 19, 2004; www.australianreview.net/digest/2004/03/harvey.html.

4

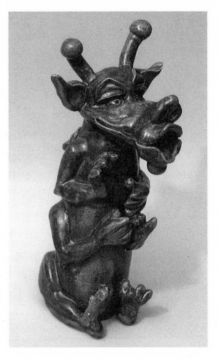

Half of all personal bankruptcies in the United States were the result of sickness and medical debt—and three-quarters of the medically bankrupt had health insurance. "They arrived at the bankruptcy courthouse exhausted and emotionally spent, brought low by a health care system that could offer physical cures but that left them financially devastated."

—ELIZABETH WARREN,
LAW PROFESSOR AT
HARVARD UNIVERSITY

Paying for Doctors and Medical Services

What Constitutes Fair Pay?

My initial investigation into pharmaceuticals had of course been merely an exercise in fiscal self-preservation—I was interested in getting enough knowledge to pay fairly but as little as possible for Patricia's medications. With the same objective, I began to look at Patricia's doctor and laboratory bills, which by this time were quite substantial. I wanted to pay these bills, but I was wondering if they were inflated in the same fashion as the bills she was getting for chemotherapy injections. If they were, then I did not want to pay the full billed amounts; instead I wanted to pay amounts that seemed proper—amounts that would adequately compensate the providers for their services, but no more. My problem was that I had not the slightest idea of what would constitute fair pay. One possibility that soon came to mind was to find out what Medicare would pay for the procedures Patricia was undergoing, and also if that level of payment was fair. If so, I could offer to pay the providers the same as they would get from Medicare.

Helping to steer me in this direction was an almost chance meeting one day with a local ophthalmologist who was treating my wife. I started discussing with him my experience with buying Patricia's chemotherapy drugs, and that led into discussion of what constituted proper payments to doctors. He made what was to me a highly meaningful comment to the effect that, under the circumstances, all of Patricia's medical providers should be willing to discount their bills to her. The billings were inflated, he implied, but he did not necessarily believe that Medicare's payments to doctors were adequate. For one thing, he said, Alaska costs were much higher, but the doctors here were being paid by Medicare at the same rates as those in Seattle. (I would later learn that he was not correct in that regard, and the realization made me aware that even those in the medical profession sometimes lack full comprehension of the financial aspects of their trade.) This man was very helpful; he even offered to have his billing personnel help me find the Medicare allowance amounts for several procedures Patricia had undergone.

And so I embarked on a study to determine how much Medicare was paying medical providers for their services, and if those payments seemed reasonable. Maybe they were not, because I was hearing that some medical practitioners were refusing to take on new Medicare patients because the practitioners thought the rates were too low. Related to that issue could be the level of payment that medical providers receive from patients not on Medicare but who have private insurance. Presumably these rates must be higher than Medicare rates, and if so, how much higher? So I was faced with several questions, and there seemed no way to do this other than to dig into the details.

One of the first things I needed to do, I realized, was to get a better grasp on exactly how the Medicare and Medicaid systems work. Being insured by Medicare myself, I knew something about the system, but clearly not enough to understand the relationship between this and other health coverage systems and their relationship to the providers of medical care. So, assuming that others might share in my limited level of comprehension, I present here a short summary of how the Medicare and Medicaid systems operate.

Medicare and Medicaid

Medicare is a federal program operated by the **Centers for Medicare and Medicaid Services (CMS)** intended to provide basic healthcare services for those aged 65 and older and certain younger disabled individuals such as those with permanent conditions or diseases such as diabetes. Medicare provides these services without regard to income level; however, beneficiaries must pay premiums, **deductibles**, and for any coinsurance. Medicare is divided into four parts:

▶ *Medicare Part A*—Part A provides hospital coverage that pays a major portion of necessary **inpatient** hospital care, and, after a hospital stay, limited inpatient care in a skilled nursing home, and also for home health care and **hospice** care.

▶ *Medicare Part B*—Part B is medical coverage that pays the major part of medically necessary hospital outpatient care and physician and related services and supplies not covered by Medicare Part A.

▶ **Medicare Part C** (also called Medicare + Choice; Medicare Advantage)—Part C is a plan under which eligible Medicare enrollees can elect to receive benefits through a **managed care program** that places the program providers at risk for delivering the health care. When instigated, it was hoped by CMS that this plan would reduce costs, but that has not proven the case, and so managed health programs are less popular now than in the 1990s.

▶ *Medicare Part D*—This relatively new program provides partial financial support to Medicare beneficiaries for buying prescription medications. A boon to the pharmaceutical and insurance industries, it requires beneficiaries to purchase insurance from private insurers, and it contains the now-infamous "doughnut hole" wherein beneficiaries must pay all cost for prescription drugs. (The program pays 75 percent of initial drug costs up to $2,250 after a $250 deductible for most seniors, but then nothing until drug expenses reach $5,100, after which the program pays 95 percent of all costs. The doughnut hole is that in-between gap.)

Medicaid is a state-operated program with major federal funding. Its purpose is to provide medical care to individuals and families of limited income and resources. Medicaid provides doctor and dental services, clinic and hospital services, nursing home and home health care, family planning services, prenatal and pediatric care, mental health care, prescription drug coverage, and optometrist services and eyeglasses. Medicare beneficiaries who qualify can also have Medicaid coverage.

Medicaid expenditures in Alaska during 2006 amounted to $960 million, with the federal government providing approximately two-thirds (58 percent in 2006) of that by a two-to-one matching of actual funds spent and an adjustment taking into account the average per capita income in the state. (The matching rate varies from state to state, ranging from 50 to 76 percent.)

By federal law, states providing Medicaid support to beneficiaries are required to seek recovery of costs from the estates of the beneficiaries. Keep this in mind if you want to apply for assistance from Medicaid. The rules vary from state to state; in Alaska, only estates larger than $75,000 are subject to Medicaid recovery claims, and some estates are exempt.[10]

Physicians' Options Regarding Medicare

Physicians are free to choose their own options for receiving—or not receiving—payment from Medicare for services provided to Medicare beneficiaries.

> ▸ *Option 1—Be a Medicare Participating Provider.* The physician can choose (year by year) to be what is called a **Medicare Participating Provider**. The physician agrees to accept 'Medicare Allowances' (the total amounts that Medicare allows to be paid for particular services). By so doing, the provider will receive 80 percent of the Medicare Allowance directly from Medicare and is allowed to collect the other 20 percent from the patients or their secondary insurers.

> ▸ *Option 2—Be a Non-participating Medicare Provider.* The physician can choose to be what is called a **Non-participating Medicare Provider**. By choosing this option, the physician accepts Medicare patients on a case-by-case basis, but will receive only 95 percent of the direct

payment awarded a Medicare Participating Provider. However, he is allowed to collect from the patient or the patient's secondary insurer an amount that will bring his total payment up to 115 percent of the Medicare Allowance. Thus, by choosing this option the physician can obtain a 15 percent higher payment for his services, but at slightly higher risk of not receiving the full amount of the higher overall payment.

▸ *Option 3—Be a Private-Pay Contractor.* The physician chooses to opt out of Medicare altogether, and he cannot bill Medicare for any services provided to any patient within the two years following the choice of this option. If a Medicare-insured patient accepts services from a **Private-Pay Contractor**, the amount he pays in full is the amount upon which the two agree, and Medicare has nothing to say about that amount, other than to require that physicians not routinely charge such patients less than the Medicare allowance for the service provided. If they do, they are in danger of running afoul of antitrust laws.[11]

The Medicare Part B Payment System

Because I was contemplating it as a possible basis for negotiating fair payment to Patricia's medical providers, it seemed imperative that I understand in detail the Medicare Part B payment system. I was soon to learn that this system's methodology is also the primary basis for the payments private insurers pay for medical services, and therefore that it has widespread application in the whole spectrum of medical finances.

Recall that Medicare Part A is a payment system for reimbursing hospitals for inpatient care, and Part B reimburses for outpatient nonhospital medical care. The Medicare Part B payment system is very complex because it attempts to take into account many factors. These include the variation across the United States in physicians' salaries, the costs of operating their offices, and the costs of malpractice insurance. By treating each of these three items separately and defining their costs in each of the one hundred so-called **Medicare Localities** in the United States, the payment system seeks to provide fair pay to providers in each locality. It is important to remember that the Medicare Part B payment structure is designed to pay not just the costs of necessary facilities and **malpractice** insurance, but also the salaries of the medical providers. It has a provision for extra pay to physicians willing to serve in certain less desirable (to them) areas of the country.

It seems fair to warn the reader that the path immediately ahead leads through a morass of concepts and numbers. Few of the concepts and none of the numbers are important by themselves, but the journey through them can at least lead to reasonable understanding and a feeling for the overwhelming complexity of the Medicare payment system.

Coding the medical procedure

The basis for determining what Medicare Part B pays for nonhospital medical services is an elaborate system called the **Health Care Common Procedure Coding System (HCPCS)** that has two parts: Level I and Level II. Level I is a coding system wherein a five-digit number is assigned to medical services primarily furnished by physicians and other healthcare professionals. The assigned numbers are called **Current Procedural Terminology (CPT)** code designations. For example, Code 71010 means chest x-ray, and Code 36430 is a blood transfusion. CPT code designations can have two different parts, one related to technical aspects (physical facilities) of the procedure and the other to the professional aspect (the labor involved). In addition to the more than 7000 CPT codes there are more than 2300 Level II HCPCS codes to identify products, supplies, and services not included in the CPT codes. Level II codes consist of a letter followed by four digits. Oddly enough, the Level I CPT codes are developed, maintained, and copyrighted by the American Medical

Association, but the Level II HCPCS codes are developed by the Center for Medicare and Medicaid Services and are in the public domain.[12] It is possible to buy books or CDs containing them. The AMA gives free use of the CPT codes to the government for use by Medicare and Medicaid, but other users must pay royalties. Just to look at the codes on the AMA's website, a patient may have to pay an annual fee of $10, and any print publisher of the codes must pay a royalty of 7.5 percent of the product's sale price. The American Medical Association reported that in 2002 it earned $71 million from CPT code royalties.[13]

Relative Value Units: rating the financial weight of a procedure

The starting point for determining payments to physicians is the **Resource-Based Relative Value Scale (RBRVS)** put into effect in 1992. In principle, it is a scheme that for each CPT code procedure generates a Medicare payment allowance that takes into account physician's time, physician's practice costs (staff, office rent, supplies), and malpractice insurance costs. The first step in the process is to establish for each CPT Code procedure the relative value of the three involved components. The result is a set of three **Relative Value Units (RVUs)** that I designate here as RVU_{WORK}, RVU_{PRAC}, and RVU_{MAL}.

Of the three Relative Value Units, RVU_{WORK} is perhaps the most complex because the setting of its value takes into account the time the physician spends on preservice, intraservice, and postservice activities. As well as the physician time required to perform each service function, the final RVU_{WORK} value accounts for the technical skill and physical effort involved, the mental effort and judgment required, and also the associated psychological stress on the physician. Committees of physicians make the relevant value decisions, and the fact that most of the committee members are specialists probably contributes to the setting of highest RVU values to procedures in which specialists are involved.

Table 4.1 - Three examples of RVU values with (in parentheses) the United States average Medicare allowance dollar amounts awarded.

CPT Code	RVU$_{WORK}$	RVU$_{PRAC}$	RVU$_{MAL}$	TOTAL
61520 (remove brain lesion)	54.76 ($2,075)	30.32 ($1,149)	10.72 ($406)	95.80 ($3,631)
96422 (chemotherapy infusion)	0.17 ($6.44)	4.83 ($183)	0.08 ($3.03)	5.08 ($192)
92004 (eye examination)	1.67 ($63.29)	0.68 ($25.77)	0.04 ($1.51)	2.39 ($90.58)

The entries in Table 4.1 illustrate quite well how it all works. High skill is required to do brain surgery, the surgeon's practice costs are high, and the malpractice risk is high, and so all three Relative Value Units for this procedure are large. Not much physician time is needed for chemotherapy infusion (he just supervises), the practice costs are moderate, and the risk is low, so the RVUs for Code 96422 have moderate to low values. An eye exam is of short duration but labor intensive, the practice cost is low, and there is little malpractice risk, hence the low values for Code 92004.

The idea at this stage is now to add these RVUs together and multiply the result by a number known as the **Uniform National Conversion Factor (UNCF)** by which Congress (not CMS) dictates exactly how much Medicare will allow for each procedure. As of January 1, 2005, the UNCF was set at $37.90. So the Medicare Allowance for CPT Code 61520 would be $37.90 x 95.80 = $3,630.82; for Code 96422, $192.53; and for Code 92004, $90.58.

However, it is not quite that simple. As the gadget salesman on television says in an excited voice, "Wait, there is more!" For one thing, the assigned RVU$_{PRAC}$ values depend on whether the procedure in question is carried out in the physician's office or clinic or in a hospital. If performed in the office or clinic, the procedure receives a higher RVU$_{PRAC}$ value because the physician's office equipment and staff is being used rather than the hospital's.

Where you are matters: factoring in geography

Also, the Resource-Based Relative Value Scale (RBRVS) system incorporates adjustments to account for varying costs of physicians, practice costs, and malpractice insurance across the country. These adjustments to the three Relative Value Units associated with each CPT code procedure are made before summing them and multiplying each sum by the Uniform National Conversion Factor.

To accomplish the adjustments, more numbers are brought into play. These numbers, called **Geographic Practice Cost Indices (GPCI)**, are the multipliers that adjust the outcome of the calculation by taking into account cost variations across the country. What I call here $GPCI_{WORK}$ is a number by which the RVU_{WORK} is multiplied to allow for the fact that physicians' salaries do vary across the United States. Likewise, RVU_{PRAC} gets multiplied by $GPCI_{PRAC}$, and RVU_{MAL} gets multiplied by $GPCI_{MAL}$ to account for geographic variation in practice costs and malpractice insurance costs, respectively. If a GCPI value equals 1, it means that no adjustment for geographical difference is required.

The overall calculation is definitely now getting messier because there are 100 different sets of Geographic Practice Cost Indices, one set for each of 100 designated areas of the country (called Medicare Localities). One locality is Alaska, one is Seattle (King County), and another the remainder of Washington state—and so it goes all around the country. At least every three years the Centers for Medicare and Medicaid Services publishes a new set of GPCI indices in the Federal Register, and anyone wishing to examine them can download the set.[14]

Just a simple little equation

This whole procedure can be described in the form of an equation, which really summarizes what is said above. The equation is:

$$Payment =$$
$$[(RVU_{WORK} \times GPCI_{WORK}) + (RVU_{PRAC} \times GPCI_{PRAC}) + (RVU_{MAL} \times GPCI_{MAL})] \; UNCF.$$

This equation is saying that the Medicare payment for a particular Current Procedural Terminology (CPT) procedure is equal to adding together the three component Relative Value Units (RVU) multiplied by their respective Geographic Practice Cost Indices (GPCI), and then multiplying that sum by the Uniform National Conversion Factor (UNCF). Simple, isn't it?

If the CPT code procedure 96422 (chemotherapy infusion) shown in Table 4.1 were to be performed in Alaska during 2003 when the UNCF was \$36.78, the calculation would be as below. At that time Alaska $GPCI_{WORK}$ equaled 1.064, $GPCI_{PRAC}$ equaled 1.172, and the $GPCI_{MAL}$ equaled 1.223, so taking the corresponding RVU values from Table 4.1, we have:

Payment = [0.17 x 1.064 + 4.83 x 1.172 + 0.08 x 1.223] \$36.78
= [0.180 + 5.66 + 0.100] \$36.78 = 5.94 x \$36.78 = \$218.47.

All it takes is a little easy math, but of course this must be done for every procedure a doctor performs.

It might appear that by going into all these intricacies regarding the RVUs and the GPCIs I am submerging the reader into unwarranted detail, but I have a point in doing so. Especially if the reader is Alaskan, he will want to hang in there a little longer. The devil really is hidden in the details, and the devil involved here sits on Capitol Hill.

An interesting anomaly comes to light when one looks over the GPCI indices published for 2003, 2004, and 2005. Starting with the 2003 set, one sees that most of the $GPCI_{WORK}$ indices for that year hover near 1.000, and in fact lie in the range 0.880 – 1.070. The range of the $GPCI_{PRAC}$ values is somewhat greater, 0.825 – 1.500. The variation in the $GPCI_{MAL}$ is vastly greater, from a low of 0.275 (in Puerto Rico) to a high of 2.738 (in Detroit, Michigan). Thus we see that the geographic variation in the direct physician labor cost is relatively small around the United States, varying not more than 12 percent from the norm.

Physician practice costs vary from 17 percent below the average to as much as 50 percent higher. By comparison, malpractice insurance costs show extreme variation. In Puerto Rico the cost of malpractice insurance is only 27.5 percent of average, but in Detroit it is 234 percent, and it is also high in the Chicago and New York City areas. (There has to be an urban lawyer joke in here somewhere.)

Here, however, the variation in malpractice cost is just an interesting side issue. The main point I wish to make comes from an examination of the array of GPCI values published each year. First, looking at the 2003 set, it is apparent that the process for establishing the CPCI values treats each of the three areas—Work, **Practice Expense**, and Malpractice Insurance—individually, and by some (we hope) impartial human-directed numerical process.* That is obvious because in no case does the process yield identical values. Table 4.2, showing the first five sets in the alphabetical listing, illustrates this point.

Table 4.2 - First 5 of 100 GPCI sets for 2003.

Locality	$GPCI_{WORK}$	$GCPI_{PRAC}$	$GPCI_{MAL}$
Alabama	0.978	0.870	0.807
Alaska	1.064	1.172	1.223
Arizona	0.994	0.978	1.111
Arkansas	0.953	0.847	0.340
Anaheim, CA	1.037	1.184	0.995

In none of these five sets do any of the two GPCIs have identical values, and that is true of all 100 sets. However, if we create a similar table (Table 4.3) for the years 2004 and 2005, a strange anomaly pops up.

Jumping off the page is that row of **1.670s** for Alaska. Clearly, the method used for determining all the 300 GPCI

---

* In fact, it is done by committee, and Dr. Alan Morris, who has participated in the process, told me that I really did not want to know what went on in these meetings, just as a person would prefer not knowing how sausage is made.

Table 4.3 - First 5 of 100 GPCI sets for 2004 and 2005.

Locality	GPCI$_{WORK}$ 2004/2005	GCPI$_{PRAC}$ 2004/2005	GPCI$_{MAL}$ 2004/2005
Alabama	1.000/1.000	0.870/0.858	0.779/0.752
Alaska	1.670/1.670	1.670/1.670	1.670/1.670
Arizona	1.000/1.000	0.978/0.985	1.090/1.069
Arkansas	1.000/1.000	0.847/0.839	0.389/0.438
Anaheim, CA	1.370/1.036	1.184/1.210	0.955/0.954

values for 2003 and the other 594 values for 2004 and 2005 was not used to determine the Alaska values for 2004 and 2005. It is obvious that the Alaska values were set by decree, and in fact that was the case. Thanks to the intervention of Alaska's pork-barreling specialist Senator Ted Stevens, Congress corrupted the system by taking the matter out of the hands of the Centers for Medicare and Medicaid Services and arbitrarily setting the values of the Alaska CPCIs at 1.67.[15,16] It was a heck of a deal for the Alaska medical providers who had obviously lobbied the senator to take this action. The amounts they previously were receiving for treating Medicare and Medicaid patients suddenly jumped 40 to 50 percent. Of course nobody else in the other 99 of the nation's Medicare Localities received a similar reward. In fact, Alaska's pork-barrel gift came directly out of their hides because it reduced the share given to each other locality.

Although I considered this action to be an example of Congress's and probably the White House's abuse of power, it left me with no doubt that the Alaska Medicare allowance was a fair basis for negotiating with Patricia's Alaska medical providers on how much they should be paid for their services. If they received that much in payment, I could be reasonably sure that none of them was going to lose money by treating Patricia. At this rate of payment her illness was not going to create a financial burden on the medical establishment or any other element of society. Bearing on that issue is the level of physician income and how it varies with the insurance status of the clientele served.

Physicians' Incomes

What happens to the money paid to a physician by Medicare? A large fraction, 40 to 55 percent, goes to compensate the physician for his own time. The second largest fraction goes to practice expense: nurses, health technologists, and administrative supporters such as billing services. Next in line are office rent costs, and approximately fourteen percent goes to medical supplies, equipment, and miscellaneous expenses. The smallest portion is for professional liability insurance, which on average runs about three percent, but in some specialties is several times that.[17] For example, a Fairbanks obstetrician/gynecologist specialist who asked that his name not be released stated to me that in 1995 his practice gross was $650,000 and the associated malpractice insurance cost was $72,000, 11 percent of the gross. This physician, practicing in a local clinic, stated that the payment he received from the clinic for his work that year was $200,000, approximately 31 percent of the gross. On average, he said, the clinic paid its physicians 35 percent of their gross income. That is well below the 55 percent fraction stated above for Medicare payments. The proportion of overall payment going to the physician depends upon the patient mix. A national survey of physicians conducted in 2003 found that, on average, the patient mix amounted to 28 percent Medicare patients, 8.3 percent Medicaid, 53 percent commercially insured patients, 5.5 percent self-pay, 0.51 percent charity care, and 2.5 percent Workers Compensation and other government.[18]

Most physicians tend to be a bit secretive about how much money they make, but some general information is available. Usually it is given in terms of median or average salaries. In 1994, the national average net income to physicians (that after the above-listed expenses were subtracted) was $186,600. Half of the physicians received less than the median $156,000, and the other half more than that amount, ten percent of them receiving net compensation in excess of $322,600, and ten percent receiving less than $78,000.[19] A lot depends on the type of practice: primary physicians are the lowest paid, and specialty physicians such as surgeons receive the most. According to a recent article in *The New Yorker*, the median income for **primary care** physicians in 2003 was $156,902, and for general surgeons, $264,375.[20] The author of this article cites one specialty surgeon whose work is so much in demand that he refuses to deal with Medicare or commercial insurers and makes over a million dollars each year—from patients who pay cash—more than ten times what commercial insurers or Medicare would pay. But of course that is an unusual example. For the medical providers dealing with privately insured patients, much less the 47 million Americans lacking any coverage, it is quite a different story.

I thought it interesting to try to estimate how well physicians would do on average if they were to treat only Medicare patients. The Medicare-allowed reimbursement for physician services depends directly upon the number of Relative Value Units assigned to the procedures the physician performs. Hence, the money he would receive in a year by treating Medicare patients only would depend on the Medicare Allowance per work RVU times the number of RVUs of work performed in that year. The average payment per RVU in the United States during 2005 was approximately $38, so one need only multiply that number by the average number of units of work performed. This methodology is in general use in the medical profession for evaluating physician income and work output.

According to one source[21] (and others give similar numbers), full-time primary care physicians typically perform 4,500 to 5,200 work RVUs per year, and specialists such as oncologists typically perform 5,000 to 5,700. One source cites a hard-working urologist as performing 8,000 work RVUs per year.[22] Assuming a 4,800-RVU workload applied only to Medicare patients and a Uniform National Conversion Factor of $38 results in a primary care physician direct salary reimbursement of $182,400 per year. The specialist performing 5,350 work RVUs per year would net $203,300 per year, and that hard-working urologist performing 8,000 work RUVs on only Medicare patients would earn $304,000 per year.

The 'average' annual income obtained of $182,400 for primary physicians treating only Medicare patients is near the $186,600 average income of all physicians cited above, but it is a bit of an apples and oranges comparison because the latter figure is for all physicians, and that includes both the lower-paid primary care physicians and the higher-paid specialty physicians. Another source, the University of California San Diego,[23] discusses this disparity in earnings, noting that specialty physicians earn almost twice as much as primary physicians working the same hours. One reason, it is suggested, is that the RVU assignments to procedures performed by primary care physicians are too low because the committees of doctors who determine the RVU values are mainly specialty physicians, more than 80 percent. An unfortunate consequence is that fewer internal medicine trainees are now choosing the primary care arena than were making that choice a few years ago (25 percent in 2004 versus 54 percent in 1998). Because of this, the wait time for seeing primary care physicians is increasing in the United States, and that results in a decline in quality of health care.

So although we hear that many doctors are choosing to avoid taking on new Medicare patients, or are refusing them altogether, the payment they get from treating Medicare patients in some cases is not really much lower than from treating privately insured patients. (Many sources indicate that the insurance payment rates paid by insurance companies are in the range of 100 percent to 130 percent of the Medicare rates.) It appears that surgeons and other specialists actually do fairly well treating Medicare patients, so they are probably less inclined to opt out than primary care physicians. When physicians do opt out, the reasons for doing so may have as much to do with their not wanting to deal with the complexities and slowness of the Medicare payment system as with direct compensation for physician work. Also, in times of rising costs, the Medicare B payment system may not keep up with increasingly high practice costs, and so even if the pay for physician work is adequate, the overall Medicare payment to the practice may be lower than what the practice would receive from treating a mix of Medicare and privately insured and uninsured patients. Losses due to uncollectible debt and pro bono services are a tiny part of the overall equation, amounting to only a few percent in most practices. And in this discussion we should keep in mind that many physicians in the United States, rather than being independent entrepreneurs, are in group practices or are salaried employees of health maintenance or other similar organizations. Also, in earning their pay, physicians often put in horrible hours, sometimes putting in duty stretches exceeding 24 hours.

The Results of Negotiations on Patricia's Bills

Not only had I been able to conclude that Alaska Medicare allowances were a reasonable basis for payment of the billings Patricia was receiving, my researches were giving me a lot more information about the medical system in this country and how its components operate. Particularly important was what I was learning about the difference between medical billings and what medical providers really expected to be paid.

In this regard, I thought particularly illuminating a passage I found on an Internet site intended to be read not by patients but rather by practicing physicians. The site, www.PhysiciansPractice. com, "The Business Web Site for Physicians," has a Questions & Answers section that in one place deals with medical billing. In answer to a question about billing definitions, it states (my emphasis in italics):

> The **charge ticket**, or **super bill**, is an internal document designed to capture information needed to bill [Medicare or insurance companies] for services rendered. *You don't have to give it to the patient.*

> However, patients do need some kind of receipt. Practices typically give the patient a copy of their charge ticket as a receipt. *But it is safer to provide them a more generic receipt.*

Why?

The practice evaluates the code on the super bill after the patient has left, and sometimes changes it, and the charge ticket contains the practice's **fee schedule**. *Those prices probably look huge to the patient who doesn't know the practice is rarely paid in full.* Either way, it's bad publicity.

Question: "What's the difference between an actual charge [**actual bill**] and the customary or reasonable charge?"

Answer: The actual charge is what you actually charge a patient for a particular service. This is usually higher than the *customary, prevailing, or reasonable* charge reimbursed by payers.

Here was a specific admission of the disconnect between actual billings and "customary, prevailing, or reasonable" reimbursements.

My task now was to determine from the actual billings Patricia was receiving what reasonable payment would amount to. My basis for determining what was reasonable was the abnormally high Alaska Medicare allowances for CPT procedures. The task was complicated by the fact that some of the 'actual billings' gave only partial information—they were not true charge tickets that the providers normally have to submit to Medicare or commercial insurance companies. The providers evidently felt that uninsured patients like Patricia did not need the information; patients should just pay the actual bills and not worry about the details. Some actual billings specified the CPT code numbers associated with the various procedures Patricia had undergone, but others did not. In the latter cases part of my task was to identify those code numbers, either by seeking the information from the providers' billing services or by determining them on my own by knowing or learning the technical name of each procedure. A helpful cross-check was to compare my determinations with wording and HCPCS Level I and II coding designations that the Washington Uniform Medical Plan (UMP)† has made available for download on its website. (With its approximately 10,000 entries, the printed download occupied 300 pages.)

For $200, I was able to purchase a CD that allowed me to determine the Alaska Medicare allowances for the Level I (CPT) procedures only, but these were the majority of the non-hospital actual billings Patricia was receiving. For the prescription drug and other Level II HCPCS code procedures I relied on other downloadable sources to obtain the Medicare allowances. I had exact numbers for the prescription drugs, but only estimates for the Alaska Medicare allowances for the other Level II items. I estimated these by assigning a multiplicative factor (1.3) to the applicable Washington state Uniform Medical Plan allowances. That probably resulted in an overestimate by 10 to 30 percent.

I was having enough trouble trying to deal with the nonhospital actual billings that I did not try to determine what the Medicare Part A allowances would amount to. For one reason, most of the hospital billings were coming from the Fairbanks Memorial Hospital and that organization agreed early on to a substantial discount to its billings to Patricia because of her low income. For another, I could see that the Medicare Part A payment system was just as complicated, or even more so, than the Medicare Part B system. However, I eventually discovered that if I had chosen to do so I could have bought a software package that would have given all the information required to determine Alaska Medicare allowances for the 7,000+ CPT code services, plus the 2,300+ Level II code services, and the 15,000+ ICD-9-CM codes used by Medicare Part A to pay for hospital services. One supplier offered this "complete hospital package" for the price of $3,795, claiming that this was the best deal on the market. (The ICD-9-CM code designation stands for the

---

† The UMP is a preferred provider organization (PPO) administered by the Washington State Health Care Authority and designed by the Public Employees Benefits Board (PEBB), and is available to public employees (active and retired) and their dependents.

International Classification of Diseases, 9th Edition, and is owned by the World Health Organization. It provides the basis for tracking and monitoring the course of diseases around the world, but has been adopted as part of the basis of the Medicare Part A payment system.)[24]

By using these various resources I was able to determine the Alaska Medicare allowances for almost all of the hospital outpatient and nonhospital HCPCS procedures and related services Patricia had received. The results in some cases were especially disturbing. In one instance Patricia received an actual billing of $1,400 for the professional component of a CPT Code 77300 procedure for which the Alaska Medicare Allowance was $53.80. She received another actual billing for the technical component of this procedure for $1,014.24. For it, the Medicare allowance was $89.24. So Patricia was billed $2,414.24 for a procedure that, were she on Medicare, would have brought only $143.03 to the providers. The combined actual billing was not just a little bit higher than the Alaska Medicare allowance, it was more than sixteen times the allowance!

This was the most outrageous actual billing Patricia had received. It is listed as a part of Table 4.4, showing ten of the larger actual billings selected from several different providers. The actual billings listed range from 2.1 to a whopping 26 times the Medicare allowance limits for Alaska.

Notice from the last row in Table 4.4 that, on average, the actual billings total for these ten procedures is about 7.4 times the total Alaska Medicare allowances, and also that in the Seattle area the payments medical providers receive from insurance companies are somewhat but not much higher than they receive from Medicare, about 122 percent. Similarly, the Alaska Medicare allowance limit for this set is 160 percent of the Seattle limit.

But the outstanding feature of Table 4.4 is that its entries demonstrate that actual billings have little bearing on reality—they are pretty much arbitrary. And of course Medicare and the private insurers could not care less what **healthcare providers** put in their actual billings because the reimbursement in most

Table 4.4 - Selected actual billings compared to Medicare and private insurance allowances in Washington State (2005 Rates).

CPT Code	Actual Billing ($)	Billing Times Alaska Medicare Allowance	Alaska Medicare Allowance ($)	Seattle Medicare Allowance ($)	UMP Washington State Private Insurance Allowance ($)
77334 Tech.	$478.00	2.20	$216.45	$142.61	$166.66
77334 Prof.	500.00	4.60	107.59	66.22	81.63
77300 Tech.	1,014.24	11.40	89.24	59.79	69.00
77300 Prof.	1,400.00	26.00	53.80	33.12	41.79
77263	3,170.00	11.30	279.10	172.05	214.28
77427	1,750.00	6.09	287.33	176.76	219.14
62310	720.00	4.24	169.61	104.30	136.54
88331 Prof	386.00	3.50	110.12	68.34	85.52
88305	366	2.12	172.78	111.59	124.39
32100	3,791	2.38	1,594.88	980.05	1,196.29
Totals	$13,575	4.40 (Aver. for Total Numbers)	$3,080.90	$1,914.83	$2,335

cases depends not on those billings but upon the Medicare rates. Not so for the uninsured patient. He is led to believe that he must pay the actual billings, and if he does not he may end up in court. If he fails to show up there, he may go to jail.

Early in 2005, I began negotiating with the various providers, offering them payment equal to the Alaska Medicare allowances. Actually, I was not dealing directly with the medical providers, but rather with billing personnel hired by the providers or by billing services working for them. In only one case was I able to talk with a provider directly, and he was extremely cooperative. In all other cases, the billing personnel effectively prevented direct contact with the physician or other person actually involved in providing medical services. At times, this situation for me was frustrating as well as time-consuming. It took more persistence and energy than a medical patient was likely to be able to muster if undergoing prolonged radiation and chemotherapy treatment such as Patricia was receiving.

To cite an example: on one of the billings to Patricia I saw what appeared to be a double charge, so I telephoned the provider's office in Fairbanks to ask about it. The person there told me that the answer to my question would have to come from the office that submitted the billing, one in Seattle. Attempts to reach the appropriate person in that office resulted in a referral to another office in Anchorage where the billing person was physically located. My question was finally answered: Yes, there was a billing error, Patricia had been billed $1,000 twice for one procedure, and so $1,000 would be deducted from her next "actual billing." (The Alaska Medicare allowance for this procedure was $107.59.)

By October 2005—nearly a year after Patricia was diagnosed with lung cancer—things were looking up. The mental strain and the debilitation of the radiation and chemotherapy treatments had made it a tough year for her; however, the treatments she had been getting seemed to have been highly successful. Her strength was returning, her hair was growing back, and her x-rays showed no sign of cancer. It seemed to be a happy medical story really, but the related fiscal story was distressing on several counts.

That story up to that time is summarized in Table 4.5, which covers the first ten months of her treatments. Patricia by then had received actual billings totaling $178,948.30. Except for the two hospitals involved, Fairbanks Memorial Hospital and Providence Hospital in Anchorage, I have not identified the cooperating medical providers by name in this table. In discussing the table entries I give all providers masculine gender, although several were female.

Provider A, a general practitioner, was crucial in the process, being the one Patricia first approached and who initiated the diagnosis and treatment process. It happened that this provider's actual bill, perhaps intentionally, was very low and in the exact amount that the provider would have received were Patricia on Medicare. No discount was called for, and we paid the bill in full.

Table 4.5 - Cancer financial status as of October 2005 (Patricia Davis accounts).

Health Provider (Billing/Med. Allowance.)	Billing to Patricia ($)	Write Down (Discount) ($)	Paid ($)	Medicare Allowance ($)	Percent Discount
Provider A (1.0)	$254	$0	$254	$254	0%
Provider B (3.25)	3,040	2,940	100	935.17	96.7%
Provider C (6.1)	23,215	19,415	3,800	3,789.74	84%
Provider D (2.2)	947.75	512.15	435.60	435.60	54%
Provider E (2.13)	1,733	919.88	813.12	813.12	53%
Provider F (3.9)	512	412	100	131.01	80.5%
Provider G Services (1.4)	18,015.68	5,347	12,668.50	12,668.50‡	29.7%
Provider G Drugs (1.9)	62,940	47,263	15,677	32,946.16§	75%
Hospital A (3.53)	56,602.87	38,699.90	17,802.87	16,035¶	68%
Hospital B (4.3)	4,297	3,147.55	1,149.25	1,000	73%
Provider H (2.2)	5,905	3,215.02	2,689.98	2,689.98	54%
Provider I (1.9)	1,486	0	771	760.12	0%
Total (average = 3.67)	$178,948.30	$121,871.50	$56,261.32	$72,458.40	
Percent of Actual Billing	100	68.1	31.4	40.5	68.1%

‡Calculated from Washington State Plan allowance. Alaska Medicare rates assumed to be 1.3 times the UMP rate, $9,745.39; hence the figure $12,668.50 which is high because there is not that much difference in the Level II HCPCS coded services.

§Abnormally high—and somewhat misleading—because it includes allowances for drugs contributed by manufacturer and uses 2004 allowances on all Taxol medications when those given during 2005 had a lower allowance.

¶Estimated allowance.

Provider B submitted an actual bill for $3,040, 3.25 times the Alaska Medicare allowance for the procedure involved, $935.17. As did other providers, Provider B received a payment of $100 early on, a sort of token payment to let each provider know that we were not deadbeats intent on ignoring debts. Then, in late April, I sent his billing service a check for $835.17 that would bring the total payment up to the Alaska Medicare allowance. Shortly afterwards, the provider telephoned me to say that he had just discovered what I was trying to do and that he was tearing up the check with the idea of accepting the initial payment of $100 as payment in full. Despite my urging him to accept the check, he refused to do so, and thereby discounted his bill by 98.7 percent. This man was going way beyond the call of duty.

Provider C's actual billing was for $23,215, an amazing 6.1 times the Alaska Medicare allowance of $3,789.74. I never met this provider, a radiation oncologist, but his billing personnel accepted as payment in full $3,800, which discounted the actual billing by 84 percent.

Providers D and E, with actual billings ranging near 2.1 times the appropriate Alaska Medicare allowances, both gave a discount commensurate with the relative magnitude of the billing, and that brought payment equal to the Medicare allowances. The discounts were about 54 percent.

Provider F with a billing of $512, 3.9 times the Alaska Medicare allowance, was offered slightly above the allowance but chose to give an even higher discount of $412, bringing the total discount to 80.5 percent

In the table, I divide Provider G's billings into two parts, service and drugs. His actual billings for services amounted to $18,015.68, only 1.4 times what I determined to be the appropriate Alaska Medicare allowances. I could not determine all of the proper Medicare allowances directly and therefore used a roundabout method based on published rates of Washington State's Universal Medical Plan (UMP) allowances adjusted by a multiplicative factor that I had derived from looking at substantial amounts of data. Provider G offered to settle his bill for less than the $12,668.50 he was paid, but I thought that not fair. The end result was a discount of 29.7 percent on this part of his billing.

The drug portion of Provider G's billing involves some complexity. One part involves the replacement of drugs described earlier, and the other comes from Provider G's intervention with pharmaceutical manufacturer Amgen, Inc., that resulted in providing free Neupogen (filgastrim), Neulasta (pegfilgrastin), and Aranesp (darbepoetin) injections for Patricia. The initial total actual billing for the drugs was $62,940, but the net cost to us only $15,677, so the effective discount was 75 percent. Because of the drug write-offs, I am fairly certain that this provider received less overall compensation than he would have were Patricia covered by Medicare.

We have paid Provider H an amount equal to the Alaska Medicare allowance, $2,689.98, on his total actual billing of $5,905, which is 2.2 times the Medicare rate. This provider did not wish to formally acknowledge a discount, but we have reached a tacit understanding regarding the $3,215.02 difference between his actual billing and the Medicare allowance. His biller obviously wanted the difference to appear as an uncollectible billing amount, so the biller would send us bills for three months and I was not to pay them. For the purpose of Table 4.5 I have listed the $3,215.02 as a discount of 54.4 percent.

Provider I was paid the amount shown in the table, $771, prior to an attempt at negotiation. This provider refused to negotiate (however, he later wrote off the remainder of this bill and others to follow during 2006).

This brings us to the two hospitals. Billings from the Fairbanks Memorial Hospital covered both inpatient and outpatient services. Thus, had Patricia been on Medicare, both Medicare Parts A and B would have been involved, Part A for the inpatient care, and Part B for the outpatient portion. For the most part I could not at the time distinguish between the two, and I did not pursue the matter because, early on, Patricia had applied to the Fairbanks Memorial Hospital for financial assistance, and that assistance had been granted. I just paid the discounted bills that the hospital presented to us. The effective result was a discount of 68 percent on its total inpatient and outpatient billing of $56,602.87.

By that time I knew that the hospital was a community-owned **nonprofit** operated by the nonprofit Banner Health Corporation based in Mesa Glendale, Arizona. That organization had stated that it gives insured patients an average discount of 61 percent, so the 68 percent discount given Patricia was nearly the average though somewhat larger. I thought then that this discount was probably somewhat smaller than the effective one that would have resulted were Patricia on Medicare, but it was at least substantial, and I had no qualms about paying what the discounted billing called for.

Late in November 2004, on an outpatient basis, Patricia underwent a PET/CT (Positron Emission Tomography/Computed Tomography) scan at Providence Hospital in Anchorage and was billed $4,297. Her request for financial assistance made in November evidently was lost, and she made two additional written requests during the ensuing months. In parallel, I initiated several communications with Providence trying to determine, without success, what Medicare would have paid for this procedure. Personnel were cooperative, but they said in mid-October 2006, almost two years later, that the information was still not yet available for the year 2004. Finally, later that month, Providence granted a discount of 73 percent on its actual billing. I assume that the $1,149.25 we paid the hospital was close to the Medicare allowance; however, this was a new procedure for which Medicare might not have allowed payment.

The result of all this is that on actual billings of $178,948.30 Patricia and I have paid the eleven providers $56,261.32. Thus, the cooperating providers have given discounts of $121,871.50, an average of 68.1 percent. Ten of the providers have received approximately what they would have gotten were Patricia on Medicare, despite the fact that their actual billings averaged more than three times that.

The lone holdout, Provider I with billings 1.9 times the Medicare allowances, has refused to negotiate. I had already paid this provider $771, slightly more than the Alaska Medicare allowance for the billed procedures, $760.12, but this provider wanted another $715 and said that it would not turn the account over to a collection agency if payments of at least $5 per month were paid. At that rate it would take twelve years to pay off the bill, and more than $100 would be spent in postage for the payments.

And so ended the first round of negotiations, which I think resulted in reasonably fair payments to most of Patricia's providers, at least a lot more than they would have received had I not entered into the situation. In the meantime I had learned a lot about medical finances and had realized that there was still much more to learn about this topic which should be of major concern to all Americans. My initial motivation had been merely to learn enough to enable me to make fair, but not excessive, payment of Patricia's medical bills, but escalation had taken place, and I now was motivated to develop as much understanding as possible about the overall healthcare system, and perhaps to pass on to others what I was learning.

One area that I had mostly ignored was the business of how hospitals are reimbursed for their services. So I dug into that.

10. Karp, Naomi, and Charles P. Sabatino, Medicaid Estate Recovery: 2004 survey of state programs and practices, AARP Public Policy Institute, 2005; http:// policycouncil.nationaljournal.com/NR/rdonlyres/9DE6D8EB-C902-41BB-9121-6711A688C60D/0/AARP_estaterecovery.pdf.

11. American College of Physicians, Establishing physician fees, ACP Online1/20/2005; www.acponline.org/hpp/phys_fees.htm.

12. Federal Register downloads, see www.archives.gov/federal-register/publications/faqs.html#faq2.

13. Pickering, Tom, Physician Billing – customers in the dark, MyHealthScore.com; www.myhealthscore.com/cpt4_opinions/ama-cpt4.html.

14. Medicare Payment Advisory Commission; www.medpac.gov/publications/other_reports/Aug03_GPCI_2pgrKH.pdf.

15. American College of Surgeons, Medicare physician fee schedule for 2004; www.facs.org/ahp/views/medicare2004.html.

16. A respected local physician verified to me that Senator Stevens pushed this through. Because of his ability to bring home the pork like this, we Alaskans often refer to him as "Uncle Ted."

17. Stephen Zuckerman and Stephanie Maxwell, Reconsidering geographic adjustments to Medicare physician fees, The Urban Institute, Contract RFP-01-03-MedPac (UI 07567-001-00), September 2004.

18. Medical Group Management Association, Cost survey report based on 2003 data, p. 40; www.mgma.com.

19. Carol J. Simon and Patricia H. Born, Physician earnings in a changing managed care environment, *Health Affairs*, Vol. 15, No. 3, 1996.

20. Atul Gawande, Piecework, medicine's money problem, *The New Yorker*, April 4, 2005, p. 44.

21. Health Resources and Services Administration, Physician supply and demand; http://bhpr.hrsa.gov/healthworkforce/reports/physiciansupplydemand/trendsin physicianproductivity.htm.

22. Findarticles, Physician Compensation Report, March 1, 2000; http://findarticles.com/p/articles/mi_m0FBW/is_1_1/ai_61933213

23. deGier, Vanessa, Income gaps between primary care and specialist physicians threaten U.S. health care, University of California, San Francisco, News release, February 19, 2007; http://pub.ucsf.edu/newsservices/releases/200702163/.

24. Fifer, Robert C., Professional coding: Parts 1, 2 and 3, *AudiologyOnline*, April 2, 2002; www.audiologyonline.com/articles.

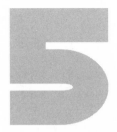

5

If we had tried to create a billing system to confuse the public, this is what we would have created.

—DICK DAVIDSON,
PRESIDENT OF THE AMERICAN
HOSPITAL ASSOCIATION

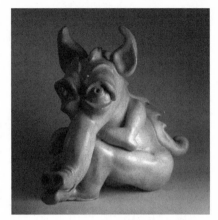

Paying For Hospitals

quickly discovered that the president of the American Hospital Association, Dick Davidson, was not kidding a bit when he spoke to *USA TODAY* about the hospital payment system. He had said, "If we had tried to create a billing system to confuse the public, this is what we would have created."[25]

No single source that I could locate offered a description of this complicated, confusing system, so what follows is what I gleaned by assembling bits and pieces from here and there. Along the way I discovered that at least 136 American universities and colleges offer advanced degrees in hospital administration,[26] of which billing and payment methodology is a part, so I was warned that this was not going to be easy. Further, it served as a strong reminder that hospitals constitute a very significant component of the American healthcare system. This general topic was also close to home because Patricia had spent several days as a hospital inpatient, and many more as an outpatient. When I compared some of her outpatient bills to Medicare allowances for the procedures undergone, I thought them very large. Even though those bills had been heavily discounted, I wondered if because of Patricia's uninsured status we might have paid more than we should have. I had no way to know except to try to determine how those billings had been generated.

Hospital Payment Methodology

American hospitals fall rather naturally into three categories: 1) government hospitals that exist to serve special segments of the population at cost, 2) nonprofit hospitals intended to serve the general community at cost, and 3) private hospitals intended to earn profit from the services they provide. Paying for the government hospitals like those of the Veterans Administration is straightforward, but paying for the nonprofit and private for-profit hospitals is a messy, complicated business.

In 2005, $600 billion—nearly a third—of the $1.9 trillion direct expenditure for health care went to hospitals. The money flows into the nonprofit and for-profit hospital systems on a **fee-for-service** basis; that is, hospitals bill for the services provided. They bill the government for services provided to Medicare and Medicaid patients, the insurance companies and **health maintenance organizations (HMOs)** or similar organizations for insured patients, and send bills directly to uninsured patients.

As an aside, I note that in the United Kingdom there is no billing at all since the government operates the hospitals, and in Canada there is no hospital billing either because the provinces negotiate to pay the hospitals **globa**lly once a year. This lack of billing expense is a major reason health care in the United Kingdom and Canada is far less expensive than in the United States—their administrative costs are much lower because they avoid the complex procedures described below.

In the United States hospitals are paid in a several ways of varying complexity, depending on the nature of the hospital and the source of payment. The simplest payment system is that involving two independent federal healthcare systems, Veterans Affairs and **TRICARE**, the Department of Defense health system serving active-duty military families and retirees. The involved government hospitals receive annual global payments (as in Canada and the United Kingdom) and the two systems provide for payment to nongovernment hospitals for needed services not supplied by the government hospitals.

Nongovernment hospitals, both for-profit and nonprofit, receive payment for services on what is essentially a fee-for-service basis. These payments are based on a variety of schemes, and virtually every payer—such as Medicare, Medicaid, **Workers Compensation**, health maintenance organizations, and commercial insurance companies—handles claims in a different way. The major payer, Medicare, pays on its own fee-for-service scheme based on averaged hospital costs. The amounts paid to hospitals are established primarily by two somewhat interrelated methodologies, one based on actual costs as determined by hospitals and government working together, and the other based on a pricing structure independently established by the hospitals and negotiated with individual payers. The latter scheme is also based on costs but may involve other factors such as level of desired operating margin or profit and a hospital's competitive relationship to other hospitals.

In 1983 the government established the Medicare (Inpatient) **Prospective Payment System (PPS)** for paying for hospital care with the idea that it would promote cost-efficient management of medical care. PPS is a fee-for-service system involving an averaged reimbursement. The system appears to be intended in principle, with its allowed 20 percent co-pays,[27] to reimburse hospitals for the full cost of serving Medicare patients and also to award a degree of compensation for more general service, in particular medical education and care for financially indigent patients. It is a complex system involving much bookkeeping.

Just as physicians and other health providers are paid by utilizing the **Health Care Common Procedure Coding System (HCPCS)** involving more than 13,000 procedural codes, the PPS system makes use of a similar coding scheme, ICD-9-CM, typically involving between 13,000 and 45,000 diagnoses and 5,000 individual procedures that can result in as many as 45,000 charge items, although most hospitals have only approximately 10,000 items on their charge structure.[28] For each hospital patient, the attending physician or other medical staffers document the diagnoses and procedures performed, and then the hospital staff codes that information into the ICD-9-CM scheme.

Each hospital or hospital chain also establishes a master schedule of charges, called a **chargemaster**, which sets the prices for each procedure in the ICD-9-CM chargeable system. The chargemaster setting process may require the work of several staffers working under the direction of a "chargemaster coordinator" and it is sufficiently complex that about 40 percent of hospitals or hospital systems hire for-profit consulting or software firms to establish and annually modify their chargemasters. As a basis for establishing pricings in the chargemaster, hospitals sometimes use cost figures or Medicare allowances multiplied by some factor. Typically, the cost or Medicare allowance is multiplied by a factor of at least three, and pharmaceutical "average wholesale prices" (AWP) are often multiplied by three or more. Local market considerations might also figure into setting the values in the chargemaster.

The chargemaster is a key document in that it sets the "sticker prices" for all services. That is, the billings that go out to all payers are fixed by the hospital chargemaster. However, the actual reimbursement a hospital receives will, in most cases, be less than called for by the chargemaster. Hospitals normally negotiate discounts from the chargemaster rates with commercial insurers. These discounts typically differ from one insurer to the next, and they can be quite substantial. Nonprofit Sutter Health, which operates a number of hospitals in northern California, states that its average contractual allowance (write-off percentage) to private insurance payers is 58 percent, and as stated earlier, nonprofit Banner Health, which operates hospitals in western states (and the Fairbanks Memorial Hospital), states its average write-off to private insurance payers is 61 percent.[29]

However, the chargemaster rates influence only peripherally the reimbursements that hospitals receive from government payers such as Medicare and Medicaid. Medicare inpatient reimbursements are determined by the Prospective Payment System (PPS) briefly described earlier, one directly employing the several thousand procedures described by the ICD-9-CM coding system. The Medicare payment system is inherently complex. The Centers for Medicare and Medicaid Services (CMS) adds even more complexity by using separate PPSs to reimburse **acute care** hospitals for their inpatient and their outpatient services, and yet others to reimburse inpatient psychiatric facilities, outpatient psychiatric facilities, **long-term care** hospitals, skilled nursing facilities, home health agencies, and hospice care.[30]

After a physician working in a hospital identifies the diagnoses and procedures performed on a patient and the hospital staff has coded that information into the ICD-9-CM scheme, the next step in the Medicare payment process is to group the coded items into one of 500+ "clinically coherent" categories called **Diagnosis Related Groups (DRGs)**. This process is performed not by the hospital but rather by an **intermediary** (also called fiscal intermediary) which is usually a for-profit insurance company that contracts with Centers for Medicare and Medicaid Services to perform such work.

All patients assigned to a Diagnosis Related Group by the intermediary are assumed to have a similar clinical condition. The Prospective Payment System then establishes payments based on the average cost of treating patients in the assigned DRG. In order to account for the unequal costs of the DRGs, each year the CMS assigns a numerical relative weight to each DRG. This assigned weight relates the cost of the DRG to the average cost of all 500+ DRGs across the nation during the previous year or accounting period. If the Diagnosis Related Group cost is exactly equal to the average, the assigned **DRG Weight** equals 1.0; if the grouping's cost is twice the average, then the numerical DRG Weight is 2.0, and so on.

The intermediary multiplies the DRG Weight by an annually adjusted **Base Payment Rate** that has been determined by federal statute and consists of labor-related and nonlabor shares. The intermediary adjusts the labor share by the wage labor index applicable to the area where the hospital is located, and applies for hospitals in Alaska and Hawaii an additional cost-of-living factor.[31] However, recently enacted law sets a common Base Payment Rate for hospitals in large urban areas.* The law establishes a procedure to set the payment rate by adjusting the previous year's rate according to set rules. The rules involve examination of a medical "market basket" and applying any percentage changes to the previous base rate. This market basket consists of two components, labor costs and capital costs, each

---

* This is the Medicare Prescription Drug, Improvement, and Modernization Act of 2003, Public Law 108-173. It is 2,065 pages long, about the same length as a modern King James Bible.

treated separately. In 2005, the Base Payment Rate (also called the Standard DRG Payment) was $4,569.83, and the combined market basket inflation was 3.7 percent. Thus, these two numbers set the 2006 Base Payment Rate at $4,738.91. (During December 2006, Congress was considering changing this formula to avoid what amounts to an enforced pay cut to hospitals.)

Perhaps it is useful at this point to examine some of the actual Diagnosis Related Groups to see how they relate to various medical conditions, the amounts charged for them, and what hospitals receive in payment. Helpful for this purpose is the recent release by the Centers for Medicare and Medicaid Services (CMS) of information on Medicare payments made to hospitals in the United States for the thirty most common elective DRG procedures. That information is given in Table 5.1 (p. 58) for twenty of these procedures, selected for inclusion here because they are performed in both Fairbanks and Anchorage hospitals. Since these are the most commonly performed procedures, the table gives a good idea of the sorts of problems many people have when they enter a hospital, and none of them sound very enjoyable for the patient. One purpose of the table is to give some idea of how various procedures are grouped into the DRG scheme, and how any complications influence the DRG assignment. When complications are present, they require placement in a separate DRG with increased weight.

The table's third column shows the DRG weights for the procedures, and the fourth the average charges for the procedures and the average actual payments received from Medicare. The last column gives the ratio of the average charge to payment. The "charge" here is the amount an uninsured patient would normally be charged, and the "pay" is the amount Medicare actually pays (80 percent of calculated cost). Notice that the average charge-to-payment ratio is in the range 2.81 to 4.49, and that the overall average is 3.20. In other words, the average billing charge to uninsured patients is 320 percent of what the United States hospitals receive on average from Medicare. The discounts given

Table 5.1 - Top national 20 elective inpatient hospital Diagnosis Related Groups (DRGs) for 2005 that are also performed in Anchorage and Fairbanks hospitals.[32]

DRG	Description	DRG Weight	National Charge/Pay (in dollars)	Ratio Nat. Ch. /Pay
149	Major Large & Small Bowel Procedures	1.33	26,523/ 8,875	2.99
154	Stomach, Esophageal & Duodenal Procedures	3.91	77,558/ 27,558	2.81
159	Hernia Procedures with Complications	0.977	27,198/ 8,548	3.12
160	Hernia Procedures without Complications	0.729	16,310/ 4,991	3.27
197	Total Cholecystectomy	2.51	47,478/ 15,369	3.09
209	Major Joint & Limb Reattachment Procedures	2.25	36,644/ 11,761	3.12
223	Major Shoulder, Elbow & other Procedures	0.783	21,942/ 6,518	3.37
303	Kidney, Ureter & Major Bladder Procedure	2.52	44,624/ 15,173	2.94
310	Transurethral Procedures with Complications	0.823	22,958/ 6,951	3.30
315	Other Kidney & Urinary Tract O.R Procedures	1.48	41,122/ 13,454	3.06
336	Transurethral Prostatectomy with Complications	0.626	18,046/ 4,017	4.49
337	Transurethral Prostatectomy W/O Complications	0.622	10,993/ 3,446	3.19
356	Female Reproductive System Reconstruction	0.674	14,008/ 4,407	3.18
359	Uterine & Adnexa Proc. for Non-malignancy	0.682	15,084/ 4,855	3.11
471	Bilateral or Major Joint Proc., Lower Extremity	4.47	56,385/ 18,685	3.12
493	Laproscopic Cholecystectomy W Complication	1.32	34,137/ 10,814	3.16
494/	Laproscopic Cholecystectomy W/O Complic.	0.807	19,314/ 5,971	3.23
499	Back & Neck Proc. Except Spinal Fusion, Comp.	1.67	26,631/ 8,731	3.05
500	Back & Neck Proc. Ex. Spinal Fus. W/O Comp.	0.899	17,541/ 5,631	3.12
520	Cervical Spinal Fusion without Complications	1.42	33,131/ 10,043	3.30
	Average Ratio of National Charges to Actual Payments			3.20

to private insurers, typically in the range 35 to 65 percent, usually result in payments higher than the Medicare payments, but still far less than the payments asked of uninsured patients.

I return now to the specifics of the payments for individual Diagnosis Related Groups. In principle, if a hospital in a large urban area were to discharge a patient in a Diagnosis Related Group with DRG Weight = 1.0 during 2006, the Medicare A payment would be $4,738.91, and if it had DRG weight = 2.0 the payment would be $4,738.91 x 2.0 = $9,677.82. However, the actual payments will usually be somewhat bigger because of technical adjustments made to account for special circumstances relating to the particular hospital. Also, the Standard DRG Payment pertains only to hospitals in large urban areas. Those hospitals in smaller population areas—specifically hospitals designated as **sole community hospitals (SCH)**—receive payment that also depends primarily on hospital-specific costs. (A sole community hospital is a hospital which is (1) more than 50 miles from any similar hospital, or (2) is the exclusive provider of services to at least 75 percent of its service area populations, or (3) has been designated as a sole community hospital (SCH) under previous rules. The Medicare Diagnosis Related Group program makes special optional payment provisions for sole community hospitals (most of which are rural), including providing that their rates are set permanently so that 75 percent of their payment is hospital-specific and only 25 percent is based on standard DRG rates. All private Alaska hospitals except those in Anchorage and Sitka are sole community hospitals.)

Adding to the complexity is that the Diagnosis Related Group payment rate for one of these sole community hospitals is based in part on summing the DRG weights of all patients discharged from that hospital divided by the number of discharges. The resulting number is called the **Case Mix Index (CMI)** and it represents the average DRG of all that hospital's patient discharges. If the case mix index is less than 1.0 it means that this hospital's patients, on average, require fewer hospital resources than average, or if the CMI is greater than 1.0 it means that the patients require more than average hospital resources.

If a hospital's Case Mix Index is less or greater than 1, a determination of its DRG = 1 cost results from dividing the average cost per patient discharge by the CMI value. This resulting calculated hospital-specific DRG = 1 cost then accounts for 75 percent of the base rate of payment awarded to the hospital by Medicare.

So at this point we have the base DRG payment that Medicare will award to hospitals for each discharged Medicare patient—a schedule for those in large urban areas with populations greater than one million, and another for others located elsewhere, in less populated areas such as in most of Alaska.

It took me some time to convince myself that I understood all this. It took even more time to comprehend the additional payments that federal law provisions allow certain hospitals. In essence, these provisions create allowances that go beyond the direct payment for health care provided to Medicare patients. That is, these payments help support hospitals in general.

One such allowance, the **Indirect Medical Education (IME)** payment, is an add-on going to those hospitals having a teaching function. The payment depends upon the resident/bed ratio in a particular **teaching hospital**. During past years (1999–2001) the IME payments added 5 to 8 percent to the Medicare reimbursement to teaching hospitals.[33]

Another adjustment, the disproportionate share payment, goes to those hospitals (called **Disproportionate Share Hospitals [DSH]**) that serve a disproportionate share of low-income patients. The payment depends upon the percentage of low-income patients served.

Complicating the situation even further is the **Outlier** payment, which has the purpose of compensating hospitals for patients requiring far greater resources than the average within their Diagnosis Related Group. The DRG base rate payment alone, structured as it is on average use of resources by the DRG group, discourages hospitals from serving abnormally expensive patients, so the outlier payment is intended to counter that discouragement.

The determination of an outlier payment is a bit complex because it depends upon a hospital's actual charge to the patient (taken from the chargemaster) as well as the hospital's cost-to-charge ratio derived from previous operations. It also depends on a threshold amount set by CMS each year. (In 2003, the per patient threshold amount was $33,560.) The formula for setting an outlier payment is:

$$\text{Outlier Payment} = (0.8)\,[(\text{actual patient charge} \times \text{cost}_p/\text{charge}_p) - (\text{DRG base payment} + \text{IME payment} + \text{DSH payment} + \text{Threshold})],$$

where $cost_p$/$charge_p$ is the ratio in effect during the last previously approved accounting period.

Expressed in words, this formula states that the outlier payment is equal to 80 percent of the extent to which the actual charge times the previously approved (by Medicare) cost-to-charge ratio exceeds the sum of the DRG base payment, the IME payment, the DSH payment, and the established threshold amount.

The cost-to-charge ratio item in this formula looks like just another innocuous term in an overly complex Medicare reimbursement calculation. However, the ratio cost/charge brings into play the chargemaster, because the "charge" in the denominator of the ratio is set by the chargemaster. Recall that the chargemaster pricing values are selected at a hospital's discretion, so they can be changed from time to time.

The kicker here is that the cost-to-charge ratio is essentially an audited hospital report that typically represents Medicare's agreed-upon value for $cost_p$/$charge_p$ as of about three years prior—it taking that long to compile and audit the numbers. If during the intervening years a hospital has markedly increased its charging rates, then the formula for the outlier payment yields a higher payment than would result if the charges had remained constant. Substantial increases in a hospital's charges not only increase outlier payments, they boost more of the hospital's patient billings into the outlier range. A side effect is that the increased charging rates make it more costly for uninsured patients to receive hospital care because they are charged and often expected to pay these higher rates.

All this is more than penny-ante because the overcharges resulting from purposely raising hospital charges to increase outlier payments are often measured in millions of dollars, even for a single hospital. For example, one hospital (Roger Williams Medical Center in Boston) was able to increase its total outlier payments from $880,000 in 1998 to $4.3 million in 1999 by making an "error" in the calculation of the hospital's 1996 cost report to Medicare, one that the fiscal intermediary failed to discover. By raising its chargemaster rates, the major for-profit hospital chain Tenet was able to increase its outlier payments from $351 million in 2002 to $763 million in 2003, totally legally, according to Tenet officials.[34] That such increases in chargemasters might be entering the realm of medical fraud has caused CMS to pursue active investigations into hospital organizations and fiscal intermediaries about their charging practices and cost-to-charge ratios.

The topic of the chargemaster and its relationship to outlier payments leads off into another awkward fiscal issue for hospitals, the provision of care to indigent patients. Acute care hospitals are required to provide such care and are allowed to discount the charges for that care under certain circumstances. However, if a discount is given, the hospital must report the full nondiscounted actual billing amount in the figures adopted to determine the hospital's cost-to-charge ratios used in determining outlier payments. My experience is that some medical billers do not fully understand the nuances involved in this complicated process, and that they sometimes use the misunderstanding to make the false claim that they cannot legally be party to negotiating discounts with uninsured patients.

Somewhat in summary

American hospitals receive payment for their services by several routes. For inpatient compensation from Medicare A and Medicaid, the Prospective Payment System (PPS) method involving Diagnosis Related Group rates determines the level of payment. Medicare and Medicaid outpatient compensation comes to hospitals in a fashion similar to that of other providers; that is, specific fee-for-service payments come from Medicare B. Payments from health maintenance organizations (HMOs), insurance companies, or other governmental or nongovernmental organizations either are based on the PPS system that makes use of DRG rates or are negotiated rates discounted from the hospital chargemaster. Uninsured patients receive billings taken directly from the chargemaster, but those billings are often discounted by one means or another (such as offering a discount for prompt cash payment) so that the discounted amount the hospital hopes to collect will depend on the ability of the uninsured patient to pay.

Alaska Hospital Charging and Reimbursement Structures

Alaska hospitals follow the above-described methodologies used throughout the nation, but significant differences appear in the numbers associated with the charging and reimbursement structures. A factor may be the generally higher than average cost of Alaska operations. Whatever the reasons, hospital healthcare costs in Alaska are approximately 30 percent higher than the national average, and the chargemasters of the Alaska hospitals reflect the higher costs.

In discussing the establishment of these rates, it is important to keep in mind the overall purpose. A nonprofit hospital needs to set its chargemaster rates at levels that allow the hospital at least to break even over the course of a year; that is, to recover all costs of operation. Nonprofits are allowed a small profit as well, as long as that profit is reinvested in the long-term operation of the facility. (For example, the nonprofit community-owned Fairbanks Memorial Hospital in Fairbanks, Alaska, sets the chargemaster at a level that allows for a hoped-for 6 percent operating margin, but in 2005 the final operating margin was but 2 percent.[35]) If it is to make money for its shareholders, a for-profit hospital must set the chargemaster at a higher level that will allow recovery of all costs plus the desired level of dividends to shareholders. For this reason, the chargemaster markup rates set by for-profit hospitals are invariably higher than those set by nonprofits.

In setting its chargemaster, a hospital needs to look at various cost categories, a major one being salaries that typically will account for more than half of the overall cost of operation. Other cost categories typically involved are operating room, supplies, and pharmaceuticals (drugs) to which multipliers are assigned to develop the overall chargemaster.

A specific example of chargemaster construction is that of the Fairbanks Memorial Hospital. Although operated by the nonprofit Banner Health hospital chain based in Arizona, this hospital develops its own chargemaster internally and uses markup multipliers that differ significantly from the average markups employed by the chain. Shown in Table 5.2 are recent Fairbanks Memorial Hospital markups in these three categories: Operating Room, 151 percent of cost; Supplies, 280 percent of cost; and Drugs, 260 percent of cost.[36, 37] Summed together these and other markups contribute to an overall chargemaster markup of 150 to 160 percent of the total Fairbanks Memorial Hospital costs, far less than the approximately 280 percent that Banner Health uses on average.

Table 5.2 - Markups of cost items to create the chargemaster (Data provided by Fairbanks Memorial Hospital and Institute for Health & Socio-economic Policy[38]).

Item	Fairbanks Markup	Alaska Average (Rank)	Highest State	Highest Markup
Operating Room	151%	156% (50)	California	450%
Drugs	260%	251% (50)	Rhode Island	937%
Supplies	280%	293% (40)	New Mexico	822%

The chargemaster computation is complicated, in part because of the difficulty of establishing the exact cost associated with each item in the multi-thousand-item final chargemaster. Further complicating the issue is the time required to determine actual costs, and so a lag often occurs between the time a service is given and the time the true cost of that service can be computed. And in some instances the rates for certain chargemaster items may be set at levels that the traffic will bear with little regard for actual costs. The end result is that—inadvertently or intentionally—some services a hospital provides will be compensated for in amounts either below or above actual costs; hospitals tend to make money on imaging procedures and on surgical cases while losing money on cases involving emergency care and chronic care of inpatients.[39] Part of the reason for the imbalance is that Medicare allowances for some service categories yield higher reimbursement rates than for others, and therefore the imbalance is outside the control of the hospital.

Because a nonprofit hospital need only set its overall chargemaster rates sufficient to recover all costs, it would seem not to matter much if some items in the chargemaster result in both over- and under-reimbursements in certain specialty areas, as long as all averages out in the end. However, such imbalances allow for-profit specialty clinics to enter the field and successfully compete with the nonprofit hospital in those areas where the chargemaster or the Medicare reimbursement does not accurately reflect actual costs. Such competition then can force the nonprofit hospital to raise its chargemaster rates in the previously under-compensated areas such as emergency room services and cardiovascular care in order to break even overall. The end result is higher overall costs for patients who then must pay not only for the higher costs of the nonprofit hospital, but also for the profit taken by the competing for-profit specialty clinics.

Sadly, the Medicare system itself contributes to the problem by paying for specific (HCPCS) procedures not according to cost but rather according to how they are delivered: a procedure performed in a hospital typically receives a different reimbursement than the same procedure performed in an ambulatory surgical center. Medicare illogically pays hospitals more than ambulatory patient centers for some procedures and less for others, sometimes by substantial amounts, exceeding 100 percent. The imbalances may in some cases create opportunities exploitable by for-profit specialty clinics, and in others work against them. Yet, because of various congressional dictates over the years, CMS has no power to address these imbalances.[40] This particular situation is one of many that lead people to view the American medical system as dysfunctional.

That all this is a matter of serious concern for those interested in reducing the cost of American health care is shown by a number of recent publications regarding the overall effects of the many physician-owned for-profit specialty clinics springing up around the country. The general conclusion is that stated above: the entry of for-profit specialty clinics is helping to drive up overall healthcare costs. Another concern is that the proliferation of physician-owned imaging clinics in particular is leading to overuse of such facilities by the owners without significantly improving health care.[41, 42]

Table 5.2 also presents the average markups in recent use for all Alaska hospitals and entries for the average markups in the highest markup states. Note that the operating room, drug, and supplies markups for Fairbanks Memorial Hospital and other Alaska hospitals are comparatively low. In fact, Alaska ranks lowest of all states in operating room and drug markups, and is also very low (40th place) in markups of supply costs.

That Alaska hospital markups are relatively low is confirmed in Table 5.3, showing the chargemaster markups over cost for a spectrum of hospitals, from the most to the least expensive. The range extends downward from a markup a few times cost to no markup at all, passing through the national average markup of 244 percent. The distinction between for-profit and nonprofit hospitals becomes quite clear here: the for-profits are at the top of the range, and the nonprofits at the bottom. And of course there is good reason for this, because the sole role of the nonprofit hospitals is to provide health care to the communities they serve on a break-even basis, whereas for-profit hospitals are in the business to make money for their investors. The higher the chargemaster markup over cost, the greater the potential for profit.[43]

Notice in Table 5.3 that the markup over cost of the Fairbanks Memorial Hospital is nearly identical to that of the highly respected Mayo Foundation hospitals; they also are nonprofits dedicated to providing full service medical care to all patients.

Table 5.3 - Chargemaster prices as percentage of costs for various hospitals or states: Data for Fiscal Year 2003/2004.[44]

Hospital	Chargemaster Price as Percent of Cost
Doctors Medical Center of Modesto (Nation's most expensive hospital, operated by for-profit Tenet Healthcare Corp.)	1,076
New York (100 most expensive for-profits)	738
Texas (100 most expensive for-profits)	700
Louisiana (100 most expensive for-profits)	651
New Jersey (100 most expensive for-profits)	638
Tenet Hospitals Average (For-profit chain)	567
Sutter Hospitals Average (nonprofit chain)	359
Alaska Regional Hospital (Anchorage, for-profit)	276
National Average All Hospitals	**244**
Banner Hospitals Average (Nonprofit chain)	241
Providence Alaska Medical Center (Anchorage Nonprofit)	209
Fairbanks Memorial Hospital (Nonprofit, Banner Operated)	153
Mayo Foundation Hospitals (Nonprofit)	152
Johns Hopkins Health System (Nonprofit)	110
New York City Health and Hospital Corp. (Nonprofit)	100

Medicare and Medicaid Payments to Alaska Hospitals

Table 5.4 (p. 68) gives information on the Medicare payments to Alaska hospitals for the same set of Diagnosis Related Groups presented in Table 5.1, and some of the data given there are repeated in the table. We see that the average Medicare payments to Alaska hospitals range from 1.11 to 1.39 times the national payments, and average 1.3 times higher. That is in line with Alaska medical costs in general.

Comparison of Medicare payments to Anchorage and Fairbanks hospitals indicates somewhat higher payment and cost in the latter. The minimum DRG group payment in Fairbanks exceeds the minimum Anchorage payment for each of the twenty DRG groups shown, and in eleven of the groups (shown in bold face in the last column of the table) it even exceeds the maximum Anchorage payment, typically by about 10 percent or even more.

Table 5.4 - 2005 Medicare payments for the twenty Diagnosis Related Groups (DRGs) in the top thirty group that are common to both Anchorage and Fairbanks hospitals and are presented in Table 5.1 above.

DRG	National Charge/Pay (in $)	All Alaska Payment Range in 25%-75% range (in $)	All AK Average Payment (in $)	Ratio AK/ Na. Aver. Payment	Anchorage Payment (in 25-75% range) (in $)			Fairbanks Payment (in 25-75% range) (in $)
					Min	Max	Aver.	
149	26,523 / 8,875	10,376–11,534	10,955	1.23	10,253	10,458	10,356	11,733
154	77,558 / 27,558	29,515–42,795	36,155	1.31	29,314	42,795	36,054	33,128–33,795
159	27,198 / 8,548	10,009–13,265	11,637	1.36	10,009	14,611	12,310	11,311
160	16,310 / 4,991	5,950–6,724	6,367	1.27	5,819	5,960	5,890	6,724
197	47,478 / 15,369	18,214–20,584	19,399	1.26	17,987	18,214	18,105	20,581–20,584
209	36,644 / 11,761	14,525–16,617	15,571	1.32	14,385	14,808	14,596	16,621
223	21,942 / 6,518	7844–10,294	9,069	1.39	7,616	10,294	8,955	8,800
303	44,624 / 15173	16,582–18,332	17,457	1.15	16,582	16,791	16,686	18,971–18,976
310	22,958 / 6,951	8,434–9,370	8,902	1.28	8,329	8,496	8,412	9,531
315	41,122 / 13,454	14,579–15,201	14,890	1.11	14,759	15,090	14,924	19,233
336	18,046 / 4,017	6,102–6,746	6,424	1.60	6,102	6,225	6,164	6,983
337	10,993 / 3,446	4,211–4,597	4,404	1.28	4,158	4,804	4,481	4,759
356	14,008 / 4,407	5,361–6,057	5,709	1.30	5,361	6,400	5,880	6,057–6,058
359	15,084 / 4,855	5,808–6,564	6,186	1.27	5,808	6,268	6,038	6,564
471	56,385 / 18,685	21,595–25,650	23,622	1.26	21,595	22,161	21,878	24,604–26,544
493	34,137 / 10,814	13,287–15,016	14,151	1.31	12,995	13,385	13,190	15,012–15,016
494	19,314 / 5,971	7,479–8,803	8,141	1.36	7,391	10,791	9,091	8,351–8,353
499	26,631 / 8,731	10,194–13,780	11,987	1.37	10,194	13,780	11,987	11,779
500	17,541 / 5,631	6,826–7,714	7,270	1.29	6,741	9,024	7,882	7,714
520	33,131 / 10,043	11,531–15,589	13,560	1.35	11,532	15,589	13,560	13,325
				1.30				

However, in eight cases (shown in italics in the last column) the Fairbanks payments are less than the average Anchorage payments. So it is a mixed bag: slightly more than half of the DRG groups are more costly to Medicare in Fairbanks, and slightly fewer than half are cheaper.

Direct hospital-to-hospital comparisons are not possible from the data in Table 5.4 because the data for the Anchorage area represents payments to three hospitals there: nonprofit Providence Alaska Medical Center, for-profit Alaska Regional, and the tribally owned quasi-governmental Alaska Native Medical Center. Because for-profit hospitals are generally more costly than nonprofits and government hospitals, it is probable that the maximum cost figures for the Anchorage area in Table 5.4 relate to Alaska Regional Hospital, but the minimum cost figures might relate to either Providence or Alaska Native Medical Center.

The 2007 hospital per diem rates paid by Alaska Medicaid to hospitals shown in Table 5.5 (p. 70) provide a more direct comparison between costs at Fairbanks Memorial Hospital, Providence Alaska Medical Center, and Alaska Regional Hospital—assuming that these daily rates relate directly to costs. The entries indicate that of the three major hospitals, the nonprofit Fairbanks Memorial Hospital costs are slightly lower than those of nonprofit Providence Alaska Medical Center, and that both are 15–20 percent lower than those of for-profit Alaska Regional Hospital.

Table 5.5 shows that the costs at the various Alaska hospitals have a wide range, as is to be expected considering the population bases served and the many remote settings. With the exception of Alaska Regional Hospital (charge to cost ratio 276 percent), the Alaska hospitals shown with that data all have charge to cost ratios below the national average of 244 percent, and we see that these have no relationship to actual costs as determined by Alaska Medicaid. Except for the new extended acute care St. Elias Specialty Hospital in Anchorage, which is in a class of its own, the table indicates that the lowest cost full-service hospital in Alaska is Fairbanks Memorial Hospital. Considering the data presented in both Tables 5.4 and 5.5 it seems fair to state that the costs of the two major nonprofit hospitals, Fairbanks Memorial Hospital and Providence Alaska Medical Center in Anchorage, are very similar.

Table 5.5 - Current Medicaid per diem payment rates effective January 1, 2007. Source: Alaska Department of Health & Human Services, Office of Rate Review.

Acute Care Hospitals & Combined Facilities	Per Diem Rate ($)	Charge as % Cost[45]
Major Hospitals		
Fairbanks Memorial Hospital, Fairbanks Nonprofit	$1,834.99	153%
Providence AK Medical Center, Anchorage Nonprofit	1,934.24	209
Alaska Regional Hospital, Anchorage For-profit (HCA)	2,395.90	276
Other Alaska Hospitals		
St. Elias Specialty Hospital, Anchorage	987.20	Unavailable
Bartlett Memorial, Juneau	1,952.60	122
Petersburg Medical Center	2,051.88	Unavailable
Ketchikan General Hospital	2,055.09	135
Central Peninsula	2,246.21	Unavailable
South Peninsula Hospital	2,378.65	106
Mat-Su Regional Medical Center (fka Valley Hospital)	2,420.86	169
Norton Sound Regional Hospital	2,506.37	Unavailable
Cordova Community Medical Center	2,678.84	Unavailable
Providence Kodiak Island Medical Center	2,835.36	116
Sitka Community Hospital	3,414.06	Unavailable
Providence Seward Medical Center/ Wesley Care Center	3,526.04	Unavailable
Wrangell Medical Center	4,235.53	Unavailable
Valdez Community Hospital	6,415.11	Unavailable

A Case Study:
Fairbanks Memorial Hospital Charging and Reimbursements

Many years ago, in the late 1960s, the only hospital available to Fairbanks area civilians was St. Joseph Hospital, operated by the Catholic Church. Patricia was born there, as was her sister Deborah, ten years later. At about that time, the hospital was run down and in danger of closure. Faced with this, the citizens of Fairbanks, after failing to pass a bond issue that would allow a new hospital to be built, invited the Lutheran Homes Society to come to Fairbanks to establish a community hospital. At a well-attended public meeting the Lutheran representative told the audience that if it wanted a new hospital, the community would have to look to itself to establish one, but Lutheran Homes Society would assist if invited. Then, under the skillful guidance of the society, the diverse elements of the community came together to establish the community-owned Fairbanks Memorial Hospital which opened in 1972, debt-free, in part because of individual contributions. At the community's invitation, Lutheran Homes Society initially operated the facility. Later, when that organization's healthcare operations combined with nonprofit Banner Health, that system continued to operate the hospital, and still does today under the auspices of the Greater Fairbanks Community Hospital Foundation which owns the facility and its associated long-term care Denali Center. With one year's notice, either party can terminate the operating agreement.

As mentioned previously, this Banner Health-operated hospital sets its own chargemaster at a level intended to do slightly better than break even, so as to allow investment in improving facilities and capabilities over time. The resulting overall chargemaster markup—153 percent of cost—is too small to allow more than minor discounting to private insurers. Although Banner-Health hospitals employ chargemaster rates (about 280 percent on average) that enable them to operate with an average 61 percent discount to private insurers, the Fairbanks Memorial Hospital is restricted to very small discounts, typically less than 4 percent to commercially insured patients. It charges uninsured patients at the full chargemaster rates, but it does allow those who pay bills immediately a discount of 5 percent, slightly more than the discount negotiated with commercial insurers. These discounts are in the range 0 to 4 percent.[46]

Using numbers presented in the hospital's 2005 annual report to the community and from a recent application for a Certificate of Need, it is possible to calculate the fraction of total income the hospital receives from the various patient categories. The result is shown in Table 5.6.

Table 5.6 shows that just over half of the recovery of total hospital operating costs comes from the commercial insurance sector; that recoveries from Medicare and Medicaid patients

Table 5.6 - Fairbanks Memorial Hospital relative reimbursements from various patient fractions. Data from hospital 2005 annual report and Fairbanks Memorial Hospital Cardiac Catheterization Laboratory Certificate of Need Application, revised January 15, 2007. Data for 2006: Mike Powers, personal communication August 15, 2007.

Patient Category	Fraction of Patients in Category	Percent Recovery Rate on Chargemaster Billing Amounts	Recovery as Percent of Total Billings	Recovery as Percent of Total Costs
Commercially Insured	36%	93%	33.5%	51.2%
Medicare	27%	43%	11.6%	17.7%
Medicaid	15%	58%	8.7%	13.3%
Native Health & Other Government	16%	75% (53% in 2006)	12.0% (8.5% in 2006)	18.4% (14.9% in 2006)
Self Pay (Uninsured)	6%	13%	0.78%	1.19%
Total	100%	-	66.5 % (63% in 2006)	102% (98.3% in 2006)

amount to just over 30 percent, and that from other government-insured patients account for most of the rest. One utility of the table is that it reveals where cost shifting occurs. In 2005, commercially insured patients constituted only 36 percent of the mix, but they paid 51 percent of the total hospital costs. Those rows of the table showing a greater fraction of patients than the portion of costs paid—namely Medicare, Medicaid, and self pay—portray a shift of their overall costs over to the commercially insured and other government patient sectors. This cost shifting is less than average for American hospitals as a whole, mainly because the Alaska population is comparatively young, and so the Medicare portion of the patient mix is low. The operating margin for the year was 2 percent, well below the target 6 percent.

Tables 5.7 and 5.8 present data on revenues and expenses for the years 2001 though 2005.

Table 5.7 - Fairbanks Memorial Hospital operating trends 2001 to 2005.[47]

Item	2001	2002	2003	2004	2005
Total Patient Charges	$136.1M	$154.2M	$161.2M	$1.773M	$187.6M
Net Operating Revenue	$96.8	$106.6	$106.0	$117.2	$120.7
Net Operating and Other Revenue	$101.7	$110.4	$111.2	$123.7	$127.5
Ratio Charges/Net	1.34	1.40	1.44	1.43	1.47
Expenditures	$99.4M	$106.0M	$113.8M	$120.0M	$124.8M
Hospital Cost Per (Adj) Day	$2,426	$2,445	$2,652	$2,766	$3,148
Revenue Per (Adj) Day	$3,170	$3,362	$3,568	$3,852	$4,347
Revenue/Cost Per Day	1.31	1.38	1.34	1.40	1.38
Inpatient/Outpatient Ratio	1.52	1.32	1.23	1.12	1.04
Charity Care as Percent of Revenue	1.02%	0.69%	1.12%	0.35%	1.34%
Bad Debt as Percent of Revenue	3.45%	3.90%	3.70%	4.10%	5.90%
Total Overall Revenue/Expenditures	1.02	1.04	0.975	1.03	1.02

Trends shown in Table 5.7 are:

- A 25-percent increase in operating revenues over the period.
- A 30-percent increase in hospital cost per adjusted day over the period.
- A significant increase in the proportion of outpatients to inpatients.
- Variable charity care from year to year, but no significant trend over the period.
- A 71-percent increase in bad debt as a percentage of revenue.
- An apparent fairly uniform operating margin with one year of loss in 2003.

However, this last conclusion requires some explanation, as is evident when viewing the hospital's expense figures presented in

Table 5.8 - Fairbanks Memorial Hospital expenses, 2001 to 2005.

Expense Item	2001 (millions)	2002 (millions)	2003 (millions)	2004 (millions)	2005 (millions)	Change 2001-2005
Salaries	$37.6	$42.7	$46.3	$51.0	$54.0	+44%
Benefits	$8.25	$11.5	$11.2	$13.1	$15.1	+83%
Supplies	$15.5	$16.8	$17.6	$19.7	$20.7	+34%
Utilities	$2.54	$2.62	$2.96	$3.56	$3.88	+53%
Basic Rent	$5.8	$6.3	$6.5	$7.4	$8.5	+57%
Additional Rent	$15.5	$6.8	$7.7	$4.5	$0	-100%
Other[†]	$13.5	$18.3	$22.4	$21.7	$23.6	+75%
Total	$99.39	$106.0	$113.8	$120.0	$124.8	+26%

† The "Other Expense" category includes everything other than salaries & benefits, direct supply expense, utilities, and rent. Other items in this category are: the Banner Health management fee, physician/professional fees, contract help, repairs and service contracts, purchased services, equipment rentals, education and travel, recruitment expense, insurance, charitable contributions, and dues and subscriptions. The three largest items—management fee, repairs, and purchased services—account for 51 percent of the "Other Expense" total. (Mike Powers, personal communication, October 22, 2007.)

Table 5.8. There, a curious anomaly appears in the row Additional Rent. All other rows show major increases in expenses from 2001 to 2005, but the 'additional rent' evidences drastic decline.

The explanation of this anomaly comes from the agreement in force between Banner Health and the Foundation as detailed in Banner Health's 2005 annual fiscal report.[48] This agreement calls for an annual rental payment that has two parts: a "Basic Rent," and an "Additional Rent" payment for the hospital facility and its associated nursing home Denali Center. The Banner report states:

> The lease obligates Banner to operate the Hospital and the Home and pay basic rent based on the fair market value per square foot for both the Hospital and the Home, adjusted annually. In exchange for rents to be paid, the lease obligates the Foundation to purchase all future equipment for the Hospital and the Home. In addition to the Basic Rent, additional rent payments are required to be made by Banner to the Foundation based on excess cash flows, net of expenses, as defined. The net effect of the additional rent payments is that Banner retains the net operating income from the Hospital and the Home up to 4.5 percent of the net operating revenue, and pays the balance of the net income to the Foundation.

The purpose of the 'basic rent' is to cover the cost of the approximate annual depreciation of the hospital facilities and equipment, and the purpose of the 'additional rent' is to cover the cost of new facilities and equipment; in essence, an investment in the future. Because the additional rent is determined by excess cash flows, it is highly variable from year to year, the amount each year depending on how much a given year's net income exceeds the basic cost of operation. The rental agreement gives the operator, Banner Health, some financial incentive, but limits the overall administrative fee Banner Health receives to 4.5 percent of net operating revenues. In 2005, the net income did not exceed the basic cost of operation, so no additional rent was paid. (In 2006, the estimated amount of the additional rent was $4.5 million, pending audit.)[49]

One consequence of this rental arrangement is that the ratio 'total overall revenue/expenditures' (listed in the bottom row of Table 5.7) always hovers near 1.0, making it appear that the hospital's operation almost breaks even each year, whereas in actuality the hospital in some years is able to put money aside for the future—as much as $15.5 million in 2001, lesser amounts in subsequent years, and none in 2005. In setting the nonprofit hospital's chargemaster, administrators compromise between providing the lowest possible cost of service and allowing for some investment in the future, several million dollars each year.[50]

This community nonprofit hospital is located in a part of the nation where medical costs are approximately 30 percent higher than average in the United States. Considering these high costs, the hospital currently appears to be providing comprehensive health care as inexpensively as possible while building for the future, and also meeting the requirement that it provide acute care to those elements of the community unable to pay for that care. The arrangement between the Greater Fairbanks Hospital Foundation and nonprofit Banner Health has served interior Alaska well over a period of many years. Banner Health brings administrative capability that the community might well not be able to otherwise provide, and Banner Health network's buying power helps to offset the cost of administration.

Fairbanks Memorial Hospital Discounting Policy

The federal government requires acute care facilities to provide care to all comers regardless of ability to pay, and to have a stated discounting policy that is applied to those uninsured persons unable to pay the full chargemaster billing amounts. Banner Health, the operator of the Fairbanks Memorial Hospital, details such a policy, and if we apply that policy to the chargemaster rate of 153 percent of cost, we get the reimbursement structure shown in Table 5.9.

There is widespread concern around the country that hospitals in general attempt to seek higher revenues for service provided to uninsured patients than from the same services provided to insured persons. That imbalance results because, although the charging structure is the same for all categories of patients—they are all charged at the rates stated in the

Table 5.9 - Banner Health expected payment policy for hospitals operated outside of Arizona with, in parentheses, estimates of reimbursements in terms of actual costs.[51,52]

Patient Status	Reimbursement in Terms of Cost
Medicare Patients	Medicare DRG Rates (80 to 100% of Cost)
Alaska Medicaid Patients	(90 to 110% of Cost)
Privately Insured Patients	96-100 % of Chargemaster Rates (~147 to 153 % of Cost)
Uninsured Patients Without Assistance	Chargemaster Rates (~153% of Cost)
Including 5% Prompt Pay Discount	(145% of Cost)
Uninsured Patients Under Banner BASIC FINANCIAL ASSISTANCE PROGRAM Having Household Income up to $125,000	Inpatient: 225 % (153/228) of Medicare Rates (120% of Cost)? ‡ Outpatient:: 75% of Chargemaster Rates (115% Cost)
Uninsured Patients Under Banner ENHANCED FINANCIAL ASSISTANCE PROGRAM: When Household Income is 150% or less of Federal Poverty Level	Free Care
When Household Income is 150% to 500% of Federal Poverty Level	Inpatient: 25% to 160% of Medicare Rates (20% - 95% Cost) Outpatient: 15% to 55% of Chargemaster Rates (23% - 84% Cost)

‡ Uncertain number—derived by using Banner average multiplied by Fairbanks markup divided by average Banner markup.

hospital chargemasters—the hospitals negotiate reimbursements from private insurers that can involve sizeable discounts. Previously I have cited the approximately 60 percent discounts awarded to private insurers by the Sutter and Banner nonprofit hospital systems. By setting average chargemaster markups at approximately 280 percent of costs, these hospital chains are able to give these very high discounts to private insurers, with the result that in many cases uninsured patients do end up paying more for hospital services than insured patients.

However, the analysis presented here suggests that the Fairbanks Memorial Hospital, because of its low chargemaster markup and its low discounting structure, seeks reimbursement from uninsured patients at virtually the same rates as from insured patients. That I was able to reach this conclusion surprised me. Furthermore, it was obvious that the hospital's discounts to Patricia had resulted in payments well below what Medicare or Medicaid would have paid were she a beneficiary. I also thought Patricia's oncologist had been underpaid, and wanting to make it right for both, I consulted with the oncologist and hospital authorities about the best way to rectify the situation. Their recommendations were to contribute to a local organization that helps low-income cancer patients and a local hospice, and that is what we did.

---

25. Appleby, Julie, Hospitals sock uninsured with much bigger bills, *USA TODAY*, February 24, 2004; www.usatoday.com/money/industries/health/2004-02-24-hospital-bills_x.htm.

26. Education Portal, Hospital administration degree; http://education-portal.com/hospital_administration_degree.html.

27. Medicare itself pays 80 percent of the allowed amounts.

28. Gerald Anderson, Witness Testimony, A review of hospital billing and collection practices, House Energy and Commerce Committee, subcommittee on Oversight and Investigations, 2123 Rayburn House Office Building, June 24, 2004.

29. Sutter Health System response to the U.S. Senate finance committee's request for information, May 25, 2005; www.sutterhealth.org/about/grassley/Grassley_Response_Section_B.pdf

30. Mike Powers (CEO and Administrator, Fairbanks Community Hospital), personal communication February 22, 2007.

31. Centers for Medicare & Medicaid Services, Acute Inpatient PPS; www.cms.hhs.gov/AcuteInpatientPPS/.

32. Centers for Medicare & Medicaid Services (Download from Top 30 Elective Inpatient Hospital DRGs, www.cms.hhs.gov/HealthCareConInit/01_Overview.asp#To www.chcpf.state.co.us/HCPF/refmat/DRG/drg1004.asp pOfPage.) DRG Weights are from the Colorado Department of Health Care Policy and Financing, www.chcpf.state.co.us/HCPF/refmat/DRG/drg1004.asp.

33. CMS; www.cms.gov/AcuteInpatientPPS/07_ime.asp.

34. The Bureau of National Affairs, Health care fraud report, Vol. 6, No. 24, December 11, 2002; www.arentfox.com/publications/index.cfm?fa=legalUpdate Disp&content_id=1119.

35. Fairbanks Memorial Hospital, 2005 Annual Report.

36. Mike Powers, personal communication, February 6, 2007.

37. Banner Health Senate testimony; www.bannerhealthgovrelations.com/home/senate+finance+response.asp.

38. Institute for Health & Socio-economic Policy, The third annual IHSP Hospital 200: the nation's most—and least—expensive hospitals, fiscal year 2003/2004; www.calnurse.org/research/pdfs/IHSP_Hospital_200_2005.pdf.

39. Mike Powers, personal communication, February 6, 2007.

40. Department of Health and Human Services, Office of the Inspector General, "Payment procedures in outpatient departments and ambulatory surgical centers," OEI-05-00-00340, January 2003; http://oig.hhs.gov/oei/reports/oei-05-00-00340.pdf

41. Unmesh Kher, *TIME Magazine*, "The Hospital Wars," December 11, 2006 Vol. 168 No. 24.

42. Lawrence C. Casalino, Kelly J. Devers and Linda R. Brewster, Focused Factories? Physician-Owned Specialty Facilities, *Outpatient Surgery*, November December 2003.

43. Institute for Health & Socio-economic Policy, The third annual IHSP Hospital 200: the nation's most—and least—expensive hospitals, fiscal year 2003/2004; www.calnurse.org/research/pdfs/IHSP_Hospital_200_2005.pdf.

44. Institute for Health & Socio-economic Policy, The third annual IHSP Hospital 200: the nation's most—and least—expensive hospitals, fiscal year 2003/2004; www.calnurse.org/research/pdfs/IHSP_Hospital_200_2005.pdf.

45. Institute for Health & Socio-economic Policy, The third annual IHSP Hospital 200: the nation's most—and least—expensive hospitals, fiscal year 2003/2004; www.calnurse.org/research/pdfs/IHSP_Hospital_200_2005.pdf.

46. Mike Powers, personal communication, February 6, 2007.

47. Fairbanks Memorial Hospital Cardiac Catheterization Laboratory Certificate of Need Application, revised January 15, 2007.

48. Banner Health and Subsidiaries Combined Financial Statements, Years Ended December 31, 2006 and 2005; www.bannerhealth.com/NR/rdonlyres/DD3E9650-00D6-4385-B12B-E96BBC4E9917/29968/2006ConsolidatedAFS.pdf.

49. Winfree, Daniel E., (Executive director of The Greater Fairbanks Community Hospital Foundation), letter to Dermot Cole (*Fairbanks Daily News-Miner*), February 13, 2007.

50. Ibid.

51. Summary of Banner Health responses to May 25, 2005 inquiry from Senate Finance Committee, Chair Senator Charles Grassley, R-Iowa; www.bannerhealthgovrelations.com.

52. 2005 FMH/DC annual report, and Banner Health response to Senator Grassley; www.bannerhealth.com/_Patients+and+Visitors/Financial+Assistance+Programs.htm.

If a politician declares that the United States has the best health care system in the world today, he or she looks clueless rather than patriotic or authoritative.

—EZEKIEL J. EMANUEL,
CHAIR OF THE DEPARTMENT OF
BIOETHICS AT THE CLINICAL
CENTER OF THE NATIONAL
INSTITUTES OF HEALTH

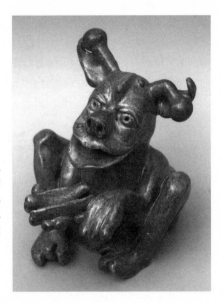

America's Health Care System

My experience in dealing with Patricia's medical bills had revealed a great deal about the complexities of the American healthcare system, but only about certain parts of it. Along the way I had talked with a number of friends and acquaintances who had encountered other sorts of frustrations, particularly in dealing with insurance companies. Some of them put questions to me that I thought I should be able to answer, but couldn't. To alleviate that situation, and for my own edification, I needed to learn much more about the workings of the overall system. For one thing, I was beginning to comprehend how big a role the financing of health care plays in the lives of a significant portion of the American population and the damage it can do to a person's sense of security. I was also recognizing that a lot of money is involved in health care, and I found myself wondering where it all comes from, where it goes, and how it gets there. My father had once told me, "If I you want to see how something involving money really works, just follow the dollar."

General Characteristics of the American Health Care System

As is shown in Table 6.1, the provision of health care in the United States is a major enterprise. In the interest of stage-setting, the first two rows of the table show the national gross domestic product and the total national debt. The United States gross domestic product is the official measure of the total output of goods and services in the U.S. economy. It is a useful number for comparing national economies and as a benchmark against which to compare various components of the U.S. economy. The mind-boggling $12-trillion number estimated for 2005 amounts to $43,000 per American. Substantial also is the total national debt, amounting to $28,000 per person.

Table 6.1 - Some comparison numbers for the year 2005, presented in decreasing order. Some numbers are estimates and so here all are rounded to two significant figures. Sources: Bureau of Economic Analysis,[53] Office of Management and Budget.[54]

Item	Amount in Billions	Percent of U.S. Gross Domestic Product	Per Capita Amount in Dollars (280 Million Americans)
United States Gross Domestic Product	$12,000	-	$43,000
United States National Debt	$7,900	66%	$28,000
Total Federal Budget	$2,500	21%	$9,000
Total National Expenditure for Health Care	$1,900	16%	$6,900
Social Security Budget	$520	4.3%	$1,900
Federal Budget for Health Care	$480	4.0%	$1,700
Department of Defense Budget	$400	3.3%	$1,400
U.S. Treasury Budget (Mostly for Interest on National Debt)	$380	3.2%	$1,400
War in Iraq and Afghanistan Budget	$100	0.83%	$360
Department of Education Budget	$57	0.68%	$290
Homeland Security Budget	$36	0.30%	$130
NASA Budget	$16	0.13%	$56

The main point of this table is to highlight the fact that health care is a major economic activity in this country. The 1.9 trillion dollars being spent on health care in 2005 amounts to 16 percent of the gross national product, and the federal expenditure consumes 19 percent of the national budget. The federal budget for health care even surpasses the war budget, and it is nearly thirty times what the country is spending on space exploration.

Now that Table 6.1 shows how the annual expenditure for health care fits in the picture of overall national expenditures, I turn to Table 6.2 to show how the money is spent. It gives expenditures for both 2002 and 2005, partly because the 2002 data are firmer than those for 2005, and partly to show the effects of rapidly rising medical costs during these past few years. The Centers for Medicare and Medicaid Services reported in 2002 that the expenditures for health care had risen 6 to 9 percent annually in recent years, a rate well above inflation, and the expenditure for prescription drugs had risen far faster yet, by 10 to 20 percent since 1999. The typical changes from 2002 to 2005 shown in Table 6.2 are similar, since a change of 24 percent over three years equals about 7.5 percent increase annually, and the 38 percent increase in prescription drug costs over the three years represents an annual increase of about 12 percent.

With the possible exception of "Nursing Homes" and "Other Medical Products sold to Public," all items in Table 6.2 show increases greater than inflation from 2002 to 2005, and two items are far greater: "**Home Care**" and "Prescription Drugs Sold to Public." An increasing proportion of the United States expenditure for health care is being spent on these two items.

Home care costs per user have risen less than a total of 6 percent over the three years,[55] so the increasing expenditure in this area evidently must be due to increasing numbers of users choosing home care over the far more expensive nursing home care. That choice, perhaps one of necessity in many cases, would explain the relatively small increase in total expenditures for nursing home care.

The other major increase is for prescription drugs sold direct to the public (excluding the drugs dispensed in hospitals), and certainly is a result of the high profits being garnered by the pharmaceutical industry in recent years.

Of the $1,560 billion directly spent for health care in 2002, hospitals, physicians, clinical services, nursing homes, and home care absorbed 59 percent, while prescription drugs and other medical supplies sold directly to the public took another 14 percent. The only other really major expenditure item is government and insurance industry administration.

Often unstated in tabulations of costs is the tax-break subsidy to business enterprises for their health insurance costs, shown at the bottom of Tables 6.2 and 6.3. This $140-billion subsidy in 2002 is significant because it adds to the $1,560-billion direct cost to bring the overall total for that year to $1,700 billion.

Table 6.2 - United States healthcare spending in 2002 and 2005. Based primarily on data given by Centers for Medicare and Medicaid Services.[56]

Item	Amount for Year 2002, in $billions	Amount for Year 2005, in $billions/% of total	Percent Increase from 2002 to 2005
Total Direct Expenditures	$1,560	$1,940	24%
Hospital Expenditures	484	589 / 30.4%	22%
Physician and Clinical Services	341	425 / 21.9%	25%
Other Professional Services	162	198 / 10.2%	22%
Nursing Homes	107	121 / 6.2%	13%
Home Care	36.5	50.0 / 2.6%	37%
Prescription Drugs Sold to Public	162	224 / 11.5%	38%
Other Medical Products Sold to Public	50.7	57.0 / 2.9%	12%
Government and Insurance Industry Administration (of Medicare & Medicaid)	106	135 / 7.0%	27%
Government Public Health Activities	51.2	63.6 / 3.3%	24%
Federal Investment in Research and Construction	59.2	74.0 / 3.8%	25%
Total Direct Expenditures	$1,560	$1,940	
Lost Income from Tax Breaks to Employers for Insurance	140	174*	24%
Total Cost of Health Care	$1,700	$2,100	24%

*Assumed to be 24 percent increase from 2002. Other sources suggest a higher figure: $200 billion.

Because of this loss of tax revenue, the public actually pays a larger share than the 35 percent stated in Table 6.3, showing where the money came from to pay for health care.

Although the table indicates no changes in the percentages with time, the sources of this information do state that changes have occurred for various reasons. Nevertheless, the table does give a general idea of how health care is currently funded in the United States. Just over one-third of the direct expenditure comes from households and other private sources, while businesses

Table 6.3 - The sources of expenditures for health care in 2002, 2003, and 2005. The rounding of most numbers to two significant places is indicative of their accuracy. Various sources[57, 58] disagree by a few percent in some instances. Percentages are assumed constant over the period 2002 to 2005.

Source of Expenditures for Health Care	Percent of Direct Expenditure	Year 2002 Amount in Billions	Year 2003 Amount in Billions	Year 2005 Amount in Billions
Total Direct Expenditure	100%	$1,560	$1,614	$1,940
Households and Personal	35%	$550	$570	$680
Private Business	26%	$410	$420	$500
Federal government	21%	$330	$340	$410
State and Local Governments	17%	$270	$280	$330
Indirect by Tax Breaks to Employers[59]		$140 Est.	$150 Est.	$170 Est.
Total Direct and Indirect		$1,700	$1,760	$2,100

pay approximately one-fourth to insure their employees and cover related costs. The rest comes from federal, state, and local governments.

The American Health Insurance Industry

The commercial health insurance industry is a major player in American health care because a major portion of the healthcare expenditures shown in Tables 6.2 and 6.3 funnel through this industry in one way or another. Health insurers sell policies to employers and individuals, and, through their roles as intermediaries and carriers, they also administer the flow of money from Medicare and Medicaid to healthcare providers. Thus, the payment for the health care received by more than 250 million people (out of a total population of approximately 300 million) channels through this industry.

Commercial health insurance is available in a variety of forms that include traditional health insurance, health maintenance organizations (HMOs), **preferred provider organizations**

(PPOs), point-of-service plans (POSs), and **exclusive provider organizations (EPOs).**[60]

Traditional health insurance allows the policy holder to see any doctor and specialist he chooses without obtaining prior approval except perhaps for checking into a hospital for nonemergency care. Policies typically require an annual deductible and also a co-payment on all services, and the insurance company then pays the remainder of the cost of services in amounts that the company determines are reasonable. The policyholder may be liable for payments on provider charges above what the insurer deems reasonable. Most policies protect from large outlays with provisions for a limit on the policyholder's out-of-pocket expenses. Policyholders usually have to file their own claims.

Health maintenance organizations (HMOs) typically cover only medical expenses from providers within the HMO organization, and may require the policyholder to choose a primary care physician who will act as a gatekeeper. Prior approval is required for entering a hospital for nonemergency services and for some other types of nonemergency care. The organization typically handles most of the paperwork involved in claims.

Point of service (POS) insurance plans are similar to HMOs but, like PPOs, allow for payment of services from providers outside the network—when the policyholder pays a higher proportion of the provider charges. Some policies limit the types of service from outside providers.

Preferred provider organizations (PPOs) are more flexible than HMOs in that the policyholder can obtain services from outside the organizational network by paying higher co-pays and perhaps taking over the task of filing claims.

Exclusive provider organizations (EPOs) are also similar to HMOs but cover expenses only for services from in-network providers, except in emergencies.

The primary difference between traditional insurance and the managed types of health care, such as HMOs, is that traditional insurance allows more freedom in choosing providers and less control over providers, whereas the other types exert significant control over both patients and providers. The latter play a dominant role in deciding what and how much health care to provide. The traditional insurers only make decisions on whom to enroll and on the amounts to be paid on claims.[61]

The health insurance industry's primary trade association, America's Health Insurance Plans (formerly the Health Insurance Association of America) claims nearly 1,300 members and says it provides health benefits to more than 200 million Americans.[62] Its members are primarily for-profit enterprises but some are considered to be nonprofits in some states, but not necessarily by the federal government. In recent years the field has become increasing dominated by large insurers such as Aetna Casualty and Life, Cigna Corporation, United Health Group, WellPoint Inc., and Humana.[63] The industry includes smaller for-profit niche enterprises like Palmetto GBA, which specializes in serving the Medicare contractor business as a Medicare intermediary and Medicare insurance carrier. With its 2,700 employees processing 119 million Medicare claims that paid $28 billion in benefits, Palmetto's 2006 revenue was $338 million, constituting nearly 11 percent of overall Medicare contractor business.[64] An extrapolation from those figures implies a total of approximately 1.8 billion Medicare claims in 2006 and $255 billion in Medicare payments, with a processing cost to Medicare of $3.1 billion, or approximately 1.2 percent.

Perhaps the best known health insurers are the 39 franchised members of the Blue Cross and Blue Shield Association who collectively insure nearly 100 million Americans in all states, and also sell secondary coverage in Canada and elsewhere.[65] The association states that the Blue Cross and Blue Shield companies currently enroll 68.5 million Americans in preferred provider organizations (PPOs), 12.9 million in traditional fee-for-service programs, 15.8 million in health maintenance organizations (HMOs), and 4.8 million in point-of-service (POS) plans. It claims that in the United States more than 90 percent of all hospitals and more than 80 percent of physicians contract with the association's members, and that the Blues System is the largest single processor of Medicare claims in the country.[66,67]

WellPoint, Inc., the largest of the Blues, and the leading health benefits company in the country, is a publicly traded shareholder-owned company. In 2006 it served more than 34 million Americans. That year it took in $52 billion in premiums, $3.5 billion in administrative fees, and $0.6 billion in other revenues, for a total of $56.9 billion. It paid out $42.2 billion in benefits to policyholders, resulting in a net income from policy sales (excluding income from administrative and other revenues) of $3.1 billion after taking out $8.9 billion in administrative and selling expenses.[68] Included in the administrative cost was $450 million in executive compensation.[69]

The difference between WellPoint's premium income and expenditure on benefits for the year was $9.8 billion, amounting to an overhead expense of 23 percent of the amount paid in benefits. That percentage is in fair agreement with a study published in 2000 stating that the overhead for commercial insurance carriers in general was near 20 percent, and the overhead for investor-owned Blues such as WellPoint was 26.5 percent. By comparison, the overhead for Medicare was 3 to 4 percent, which apparently includes the cost of claim processing by intermediaries and carriers.[70] The overall cost of administering the United States healthcare system has been estimated as amounting to 31 percent, based on 1999 data,[71] and it appears that the overhead expense and shareholder earnings of for-profit health insurers accounts for a substantial portion of that amount.

For-profit insurers such as WellPoint are involved in various activities related to selling health insurance, including loaning money and investing money collected from premiums. However, the primary source of income to the health insurance business is the premium payment that individuals or employers make for healthcare coverage. In 2006 the average annual premium paid by employers for insurance coverage was $4,200 for a single employee and $11,500 for a family of four.[72] The gross earnings for a full-time, minimum wage worker that year were $10,712. The premium for a family of four in 2006 was even higher, increasing 7.7 percent from 2005, twice the inflation rate. Since 2000, the cost of premiums has risen four times faster than workers' salaries, average employee contributions to employer-sponsored health insurance have increased 143 percent, and the average out-of-pocket costs of deductibles, co-payments and co-insurance for physician and hospital visits rose 115 percent.[73]

While these costs were increasing, the industry was consolidating. More than 400 mergers involving health insurers and managed care organizations took place between 1995 and 2005, and five of the largest health insurance companies now control 60 percent of the market.[74] Profits and profit margins have also risen. In July 2007, one of the major companies, Humana Inc., reported that its second-quarter profits more than doubled from a year earlier on the strength of improved cost controls and higher income from its government business because of the enactment of the Medicare Prescription Drug Improvement and Modernization Act of 2003.[75] The combined net profit of the six top health insurance companies was more than $10 billion in 2006.[76]

Of course the primary objective of for-profit health insurance companies is to make a profit, and they seek to improve profits in several ways. One is to lower risk by refusing to insure persons likely to incur high medical expenses, especially those with pre-existing medical conditions. In 2004, the Public Health Service estimated that about two million Americans had been denied insurance for this reason.[77] Many states, including Alaska, have established insurance programs that insure such persons at costs ranging from 125 to 250 percent that of traditional insurance, the high-risk pool insurance being managed by commercial insurers such as Blue Cross.

The fundamental idea of insurance is to spread the cost of a loss incurred by individuals over a larger population, typically referred to as a "risk pool," each member of the risk pool sharing in the cost of the loss equally or perhaps according to ability to pay. Virtually all modern nations (the United States excepted) essentially place their entire populations into a single health insurance pool and have that pool share in the overall cost of health care according to ability to pay, making use of taxation or other mechanisms. In the United States we have a much more complicated system of paying for health care—and many, many risk pools, plus 47 million Americans without insurance.

For the purpose of discussion, we can think of those 47 million as constituting yet another risk pool. In the United States, the members of any one risk pool do not necessarily pay for the overall cost of their risk pool, and the costs incurred by some of the risk pools may be borne by the population as a whole. The Medicare, Medicaid, Veterans Administration, and the military TRICARE pools are examples of that. Part of the health care required by the uninsured pool is cost-shifted to other pools, and part of the cost is borne directly by the individual users. Complicating things even more is that the memberships of the various pools are fluid: as most people reach 65 they automatically shift into the Medicare pool. Changing financial situations or changes in location can shift people in and out of the 50+ state Medicaid pools, and changes in medical condition can shift them from one commercial insurance risk pool to another or shunt them off into the uninsured pool.

One measurable characteristic of the various risk pools is their **medical loss ratio**, the portion of money paid into the pool that actually goes to paying for medical benefits. The Medicare medical loss ratio is about 96 to 97 percent, meaning that 96 to 97 percent of the money going into the program goes to pay for health care. By contrast, the typical medical loss ratio of a commercial preferred provider organization is about 73 percent—nearly one-third going for administration and profit, according to one consumer organization,[78] and, even worse, the medical loss ratio of many individual health insurance policies is a lowly 45 percent.

For-profit insurance companies know all about the medical version of the **"eighty-twenty (80/20)"** (also **"20/80")** **rule**, stating that 20 percent of the population will account for 80 percent of expenses, and they make use of it in striving to lower their medical loss ratios. They seek to insure those 80 percent of customers who need the least health care while avoiding the 20 percent likely to incur high costs, or placing them in high-risk pools to which they can charge higher premiums. The companies spend much effort—and administrative cost—in such cherry-picking activity. They generate a variety of cost-adjusted policy options, each with its own administrative rules that make comparison between plans a nightmare for consumers, and also give healthcare providers headaches trying to fill out the required multiple, differing versions of claim applications.

In such complexity lies much potential for profit—and opportunity for the inventive insurance industry to generate more complexity. This is marketplace medicine in action at its finest.

Another way to maintain profits is to minimize the size of actual payouts in benefits, "losses" in the parlance of the industry. One consequence is that many Americans are becoming increasing frustrated and financially distressed by what they consider to be insurance company stinginess. Anecdotal examples abound, and I have a few of my own that illustrate how the companies operate to try to minimize their "losses;" that is, to lower their medical loss ratios.

- ▶ Anecdote #1—A friend works for a company in Idaho that sells malpractice insurance. Her company recently changed the carrier for its employee health insurance, assuring the employees that there would be no change in cost or coverage. Not so, it turns out. A fellow employee has a special-needs child whose health care was entirely covered by the former insurer. The new insurer refuses that coverage, and so the family is stuck with an additional outlay of $17,000 per year to cover the child's health needs. The onus is now on the family to try to prove that an insurer should pay for this care.

▶ Anecdote #2—My married granddaughter with one child teaches in the Anchorage public schools. She thought she was fully covered by the policy obtained through her teachers' union. Big surprise, however, when nine months ago she delivered twin girls, slightly prematurely. Everything was basically normal, but since twin births were involved and complications could occur, the medics decreed that the delivery be in a surgery rather than a usual birthing room. "The room was full of people," my granddaughter said, "surgeons, nursing teams for each baby, and many others—and I got a bill from every one of them." During the first few days of their lives the two girls racked up huge medical bills, on the order of $100,000, and the first complication came when the insurance carrier initially refused to cover the cost because the girls were not named on the policy. This was so ridiculous that the company soon backed off on that. But this was just the beginning. Two births from one woman in one day were one too many as far as the insurance company was concerned, and confusion reigned from then on. It involved switching costs attributable to one baby to the other in order to minimize payout, and also refusal to pay some of the physician charges because they were, according to the insurer, not reasonable and customary. The insurer asked our granddaughter and her husband to prove that the denied costs were acceptable, and, as time went on, the frustration rose to such a level and the effort required to fight the insurance company was so great that the couple threw up their hands and decided to pay the unallowed bills of approximately $20,000 themselves. That amount has driven them out of the class of fully insured into the class of the underinsured (by definition, those people with out-of-pocket healthcare costs exceeding 10 percent of income).

> ► Anecdote # 3—A fully insured friend in Georgia who is a professional counselor sustained damage to his spinal column while renovating his house and became permanently disabled. His employer continued to pay a substantial portion of his salary but required him to apply for Medicare. He did and was accepted, at which point his disability insurer became the secondary carrier. The insurance company paid the bills for a time but recently informed him that they would terminate payments because the company deemed him no longer disabled. While seeking legal advice on how to deal with the insurance company, the man learned from a lawyer specializing in such matters that it is common practice for insurance companies in cases like this to pay benefits for a few years and then begin harassing the policyholder to prove he is still disabled. As part of the process the companies offer a small settlement that almost all people accept, and the insurer thereby cuts its "losses."

In each of these three anecdotes, it is clear that, by demanding that the policyholder prove payment should be made, it is the intent of the insurer to wear him or her down to the point of giving up. It works because the policyholders are so ill or become so frustrated that they no longer wish to fight. Too often they are in a disadvantaged position because their employers are the purchasers of the insurance and the individual policyholders and the healthcare providers who serve them are merely bystander irritants to the main players in this marketplace: the employers and the for-profit insurance companies.

The United States and Alaska
Consumers of Health Care

American consumers of health care can be categorized into three major groups: those having health insurance provided by Medicare and Medicaid or other public programs, those having insurance purchased by themselves or their employers from the insurance industry, and those without insurance. Table 6.4 shows the population in each group for Alaska and the United States as a whole during 2004–05. Because the population is younger, Alaska has a smaller percentage of persons with Medicare than in the United States as a whole, and a somewhat higher percentage with Medicaid coverage. Otherwise, the percentages are roughly the same in Alaska and the United States. In both, well over half of healthcare consumers have coverage purchased from the for-profit insurance industry, and 25 to 30 percent are covered by public insurance. In both Alaska and the United States, one in six persons, 16 to 17 percent of the population, has no insurance.

All people age 65 and over and younger ones with serious long-term medical conditions qualify for Medicare and, if their income is very low, they may qualify for Medicaid as well. In 2004–05, 31,000 Alaskans were in this dual-coverage situation. Others qualifying for Medicaid are persons having no possessions other than a home and automobile, and very low income—less than a few hundred dollars per month.

Insured people may have policies partly or wholly paid for by their employers, or that they have purchased themselves. In either case, the insurance generally does not cover all costs nor,

Table 6.4 - Alaska and United States population distributed by health insurance status, state data for 2004–05.[79]

Insurance Status	Alaska	% of Alaska Population	United States	% of U.S. Population
Medicare	55,600*	8.4	35,000,000	12
Medicaid	106,000*	16	38,000,000	13
Other Public (Military & Other)	33,000	5	3,000,000	1
Employer Insured	343,000	52	153,000,000	54
Individual Insured	26,400	4	15,000,000	5
Uninsured	114,000	17	47,000,000	16
Total Population1	660,000	100	295,000,000	100

*Approximately 31,000 Alaskans have dual Medicare and Medicaid insurance.

depending on the policy, does it cover all the types of medical care that may be required. The purchaser typically is responsible for a portion of the cost (his deductible plus a fraction of the full cost up to some limit called the **out-of-pocket maximum**), but if the care received is not covered by the policy, the individual must bear the full cost. These out-of–pocket expenses may be sufficiently large that an insured person falls into the underinsured category, a grouping that includes approximately one in five insured Americans. The underinsured are usually defined as those whose medical expenses exceed 10 percent of their income, or, if of low income, 5 percent.[80] An example is my teaching granddaughter whose costly delivery of twin girls (cited above) threw the family into the underinsured category.

Almost three out of four underinsured American adults are low income.[81] The underinsured tend to skimp on health care by failing to fill prescriptions, skipping tests and followup care, and forgoing treatment from specialists. Their numbers are now increasing because of the current trend for employers to shift more of the fiscal burden of health care to employees and Bush administration efforts to encourage more "consumer-driven" health care. No fine line distinguishes the underinsured and the uninsured.

Most people listed in the 47 million-strong uninsured category have low income, but increasing numbers of moderate- to middle-income adults are now uninsured. A recent study has shown that within this moderate- to middle-income group 41 percent did not have health insurance during at least a part of 2005, up from 21 percent in 2001.[82] Most uninsured people are in working families, and most of these families have at least one person working full time.

In Alaska, those people most likely to be uninsured are the self-employed, seasonal workers, part-time workers, persons working for small firms, or Alaska Natives. More than half of the Alaska uninsured are employed. Approximately one-third of young adults, those aged 18 to 24, are uninsured. Sixty-two percent of the uninsured in Alaska are Caucasian, 19 percent are Alaska Native, 6 percent are Asian, 2 percent are African American, and 11 percent are of mixed race. Although Alaska Natives constitute only 16 percent of the population, they still account for a significant portion of the uninsured, despite the fact that if they belong to a federally recognized tribe they are eligible for health care provided by the Indian Health Service, mostly or all through Native corporations.[83, 84]

In 2006, 20.5 percent of the uninsured in Alaska had household incomes less than $5,000, 21.1 percent were in the range $5,000 to $25,000, 15.8 percent in the range $25,000 to $35,000, 19.8 percent in the range $35,000 to $50,000, 12.8 percent in the range $50,000 to $75,000, and 10.3 percent with household incomes above $75,000.[85]

These data show that many Alaskans, regardless of income level, are in a precarious position with regard to paying for health care, as are many elsewhere in the United States. Only the rich—those with several million dollars in resources—are fully immune from worry that they might incur bankrupting medical expenses. Most Americans will be lucky enough to remain sufficiently healthy throughout their lives that they will not have serious problems with funding their medical care. However, the medical version of the 80/20 rule dictates that a significant number will not be lucky, and, unfortunately, the ratio of unlucky to lucky is now on the rise due to insurance companies' efforts to lower their own risk.

How the Multiple-Payer Health Care System Works

As Table 6.3 implies, we have in the United States a multipayer system: the money paid to those directly involved in providing health services—the hospitals, clinics, physicians, nurses, laboratory technicians, and nursing aides—comes to them from several sources, by several routes, and at levels of payment that depend on the route. Because the levels of payment differ, the American system does not qualify as an **all-payer system** wherein every payer pays uniform prices for medical services. All developed western countries except the United States have either single-payer or all-payer systems.

Route 1—Uninsured patient medical provider

The simplest route is the one described earlier: the hospital or other provider seeks payment only from an uninsured person like Patricia. The provider's billing personnel, or personnel employed by a for-profit billing service, prepare an actual bill that is sent to the person directly. This bill will be in an amount typically two or more times what the provider expects to be paid were the recipient covered by Medicare, Medicaid, or a commercial insurer. The person receiving the actual bill might pay it in full or he might negotiate the bill as was done in Patricia's case. If the negotiation fails and the recipient is unable to pay the bill right away, the provider is likely to accept small payments over a long period—sometimes for the lifetime of the patient. Describing that situation to me, one physician said, "Neither the patient nor I are likely to live long enough for the bill to be paid off." If the patient has a chronic condition or for other reason requires extensive medical care, he probably will remain in debt for the rest of his life. He then has fallen into what the authors of a recent book, *Uninsured in America: Life and death in the land of opportunity*[86] call the Death Spiral. The patient will never escape this financial black hole.

Temporary reprieve might come by the patient's declaring bankruptcy, as many have. In fact, it is generally acknowledged that half of all individual bankruptcies are now due to medical payment problems. If the patient has a house and a car those items will be exempt, but any other assets will be gone. Should the uninsured patient neither declare bankruptcy nor make any payments at all, the provider might write off all or a portion of the bill by declaring the billed service a "charitable contribution." (The federal government requires not-for-profit hospitals to provide some charity care, so such write-offs qualify.) Alternatively, the provider may bill the patient for the full amount and then, after sixty days, sell the account to a collection agency for ten to fifteen cents on the dollar.[87] (Sometimes these accounts are bundled into larger debt portfolios that are marketed for as little as five cents on the dollar.)

Herein may lie one reason why many medical providers set their actual billings at several times what are considered to be "customary, prevailing, or reasonable" rates. An unusually high billing will not affect what the provider receives from Medicare, Medicaid, or insurance companies, but it will raise the amount received by selling unpaid accounts to collection agencies. If an actual billing is six times the Medicare rate, and the provider can sell the account for fifteen cents on the dollar, he will receive 90 percent of what he would have received if the patient were on Medicare. In either of these approaches, it is win-win for the provider and lose-lose for the uninsured patient. If the patient dies before paying off the bill, there is a chance that the provider can collect the full billing from the patient's estate. However it works out, this is the simplest and most direct way to route money from the payer to the medical provider. Note that, even here, a portion of the money paid to the medical provider is siphoned off to pay for the medical billing services and collection agencies. If things get messy, court expenses and lawyer fees may take a cut as well.

In Alaska, we have a unique situation that allows providers to seek payment of unpaid bills by filing lawsuits to garnish Alaska Permanent Fund dividends, the annual payouts ($1,654 in 2007[88]) most Alaskans receive from the permanent fund, currently with $39 billion in holdings.[89] During the period 2000 through June 2005, Banner Health, the operator of the Fairbanks Community Hospital, filed 2,914 of these suits.[90]

Route 2—Payments to medical providers by patients with traditional insurance (not Health Savings Accounts; see Route 3)

As with the uninsured patients, the payment process starts when the provider's billing personnel or his hired billing service prepares an actual bill. That bill will require a determination of the billing code to be applied to each procedure and perhaps a justification for why the procedure was given. The bill goes to the patient's insurance company and perhaps also to the patient. Insurance company personnel examine the bill for errors and may debate the assigned coding. It is to the insurance company's advantage to "down-code" the billing if possible; that is, to assign a less expensive code to the procedure. If errors are found or down-coding occurs, the bill is then returned to the provider's billing personnel as often as necessary until an agreement is reached. This process might take several months, and additional delay may occur if more than one insurance company is involved, such as might be the case if the treatment stemmed from an auto accident involving multiple liability.

The next step in the process is to make payment to the medical provider. Prior negotiation between the insurance company and the medical provider may determine how much is to be paid. That negotiation often uses the Medicare rates as a basis, and it might result in payment 100 to 130 percent of the Medicare rate. Another method is to base payment on what is deemed by the insurance company to be the "usual, reasonable and customary" charges for services as determined by the company. For example, Employment Benefit Management Services, Inc. (EBMS), which operates a self-insurance plan for a teachers' organization in Alaska (The NEA-Alaska Health Plan) states that the maximum it pays for a particular service is equal to what 90 percent of the doctors in some unspecified database charge for that service. EBMS also states that it uses "aggressive fee negotiations with providers," that "allow aggressive discounts."[91] It receives a 35 percent discount from the Providence not-for-profit hospital in Anchorage.[92]

However it is determined, the amount paid will often be far less than the amount called for in the actual bill, unless a previous agreement has been reached between the insurance company and the provider for billings to equal agreed-upon amounts. The insurance policy involved may require a co-payment from the patient and may also demand a deductible that the patient must pay before the insurance company payment cuts in. In some cases the provider may require the patient to cough up the deductible, the co-payment, or even the full actual billing payment at the time the service is rendered. The idea then is that the insurance company will send payment to the insured person rather than to the provider, and that the provider might have to refund some payment to the insured person if he has paid more than the amount negotiated between the insurance company and the provider. The money the insurance company pays the provider comes from premiums paid by the patient's employer or perhaps from the patient himself. Again, a substantial portion of that money, 20 to 30 percent, goes into insurance company administrative costs and profit for shareholders, so cannot reach the medical provider.

Private insurance companies may disallow payment for some services altogether, and in those instances the insured patient falls into the same situation as the uninsured patient: he must deal with the provider directly and pay the full or discounted billing amounts directly to the provider.

Route 3—Payments to medical providers by patients with tax-favored Health Savings Accounts

A provision of the 2003 Medicare Prescription Drug Improvement and Modernization Act of 2003 established tax-favored **Health Savings Accounts (HSAs)**. Proponents argued that HSAs were a solution to the problem of rapidly rising healthcare costs and a means to reduce the number of uninsured Americans. The underlying philosophy is embodied in the concept of **consumer-driven health care**, which is based on the idea that if consumers play a greater role (take more personal responsibility) in choosing how to spend their healthcare dollars, they will exercise choices that will hold healthcare costs down.

They would shop around for medical bargains and consume less health care and supplies.* Another motivation less often mentioned by proponents is that HSAs shift financial risk from employers to employees, thereby reducing the costs of employee benefits to the employers.

Employees with traditional employer-sponsored insurance are encouraged to shift over to Health Savings Accounts by being allowed to place pretax dollars (limited to $2,700 and $5,450 for singles and families, respectively, in 2006) into the accounts, which they can spend tax-free for any legitimate medical expenses the account holder chooses. That includes prescription drugs and dental, ear and eye care that might not be covered by a traditional insurance plan. However, to establish an HSA, a consumer must purchase a **High-Deductible Health Plan (HDHP)**, typically cheaper than traditional health insurance by 30 to 50 percent. The HDHP annual deductible must be at least $1,000 for an individual and $2,000 for a family. The annual out-of-pocket expense (including co-pays and deductibles) must not exceed (in 2006) $5,250 for an individual and $10,500 for a family. If the purchaser is employed, his employer might pay for a portion or all of the HDHP, and might also contribute funds to the HSA.

To encourage HSA holders to seek **preventive** medical care (annual physicals, immunization and screening services) HDHPs typically have a "first dollar" provision that pays for these services up to a limit, perhaps $300. Thereafter, the HSA holder pays for everything until the limiting HDHP deductible is reached. At that point the HDHP payments kick in, paying perhaps 80 percent of expenses provided by plan-approved providers (in-network providers), or 60 percent of payments to other, out-of-network providers. Later, when the maximum out-of-pocket limit is achieved, the HDHP is required to pay

---

* That idea conjures up several scenarios in my mind. One: Man comes into house from his woodshop and says to wife, "Dear, I just cut my finger off with the table saw. Would you please call around and find out which hospital has the cheapest emergency room rates?" Another: Wife to husband, "Dear, it's Saturday; let's go shopping for medical deals and see if any of the doctors are having special sales."

100 percent up to some lifetime limit, typically several million dollars, but sometimes far less.

So providers to people with health savings accounts usually receive direct payment from the holder's high-deductible health plan policy for annual physicals, immunization and the like, up to a limit of several hundred dollars. After that, the consumer directly pays for provider services until he has spent an amount equal to the policy's deductible, typically $1,000 or $2,000 each year. Thereafter, pay comes to the provider both from the high-deductible health plan and the patient in proportions determined by the policy wording and the provider's status as either a plan-participating (in-network) provider or a nonparticipating plan (out-of-network) provider—until such time as the single patient has expended $5,250, or if a family member, $10,500. During the remainder of the year the provider receives all payment from the insurer issuing the high-deductible health plan policy. At the onset of a new year, it starts all over again.

Providers to health savings account holders appear to face a complex reimbursement situation, one that depends on the patient's ever-changing status with regard to his high-deductible health plan's deductible and out-of-pocket limitations. That situation complicates the provider's bookkeeping, and if under- or overpayments are made, they require later adjustment.

Route 4—Payments to providers of patients enrolled in Medicare or Medicaid

As in Routes 1 and 2, the provider's billing operation starts the process by preparing billing statements. These must meet the requirements imposed by the Centers for Medicare and Medicaid Services, and must be on an approved form to be submitted in paper or electronic format. Filling out the form looks to be only slightly more complicated than filling out a basic IRS income tax Form 1040. On the claim form, non-hospital providers must identify the CPT codes for physician services provided and the

HCPCS codes that represent procedures, supplies, products, and services not covered by CPT codes, plus other information relating to the patient and the procedures performed. One indication of the complexity is that providers are allowed to submit claims as much as fifteen to twenty-seven months after the date of service, depending on circumstances. Speed is not of the essence in this business.

The medical provider giving services covered by Medicare Part B submits the completed billing to what is called a **Medicare carrier**, while hospitals submit Medicare Part A billings to what are called Medicare intermediaries. The Medicare carriers and intermediaries are for-profit insurance companies that have contracted with the Centers for Medicare and Medicaid Services to process claims and make many payments, although Medicare Part A pays many hospitals directly once the claims are processed. Sitting somewhat on the side overlooking this process in each state is a **Peer Review Organization** composed of practicing doctors and other professionals that sets standards and may deny payments to providers for services not deemed medically necessary.

Complications can arise when the patient is 65 or over and thus is covered by Medicare but is working for an employer with twenty or more employees who provides healthcare benefits, or if a spouse is covered by private insurance. In these situations Medicare becomes the secondary insurer and pays only after the private insurer has done so.[93] Also the person insured by Medicare may be covered by insurance he or his past employer has purchased to cover expenses not covered by Medicare, holding what is often referred to as a **medigap policy**. The result of all this is that the payment to the provider may actually come from three different sources: Medicare, the private insurance company, and the patient because he has a co-pay or deductible. Medicaid operates in much the same way except that the allowances may be somewhat smaller and are governed by the dictates of state legislatures.

Route 5—Payments to providers for patients enrolled in health maintenance organizations (HMOs), preferred provider organizations (PPOs), private fee-for-service plans (PFFSs)

A patient eligible for Medicare Parts A and B can opt out of that coverage into Medicare Part C and join one of the HMO, PPO, or **private fee-for-service (PFFS)** plans that have contracted with the Centers for Medicare and Medicaid service to provide health care. In 2005, approximately 12 percent of Medicare beneficiaries were enrolled in these so-called **Medicare Advantage** (formerly called Medicare + Choice) plans, the other 88 percent having the traditional Part A and Part B fee-for-service Medicare coverage.[94] Additionally, about half of all employees now are enrolled in HMOs, prepaying monthly for their medical care. For their enrollees also on Medicare, these organizations draw from the Centers for Medicare and Medicaid payments roughly equivalent to what the centers would pay for conventionally enrolled patients. These organizations pay medical providers in one of three ways: on direct salary, according to the number of enrollees served, or for each service provided.

The managed health organizations—sort of combined insurance and healthcare systems all in one—began coming into vogue in the 1970s and they gained in popularity until, in 1996, more than 600 of them existed nationwide.[95] These plans were touted as possibly offering wider choice in health care and cheaper and more comprehensive care than other forms of insurance. They didn't, and soon disenchantment with them set in, and by 2005 only 247 were in operation (none in Alaska). The profit motive was taking its toll and serious question was developing about the quality of and restrictions on the health care being provided.[96] In recent years, managed healthcare organizations have sought to operate only in the more profitable regions of the country, often to the disadvantage of people in low-population areas. Providers who serve these organizations may in some cases be directly employed by the organization, but mostly they receive payment on a fee-for-service basis.

Route 6—Payments to providers to Veterans Administration, TRICARE, and similar government health care systems

Most of the health care for veterans, active military personnel and dependents is in facilities owned and operated by various government organizations, and by providers who are directly employed by them. Income to such providers is through salaries, rather than on the fee-for-service basis prevalent in the United States. However, agencies such as the Veterans Administration do occasionally go outside their own organizations for healthcare services and then usually pay on a fee-for-service basis—typically at rates established by the organizations themselves or by negotiated agreements.

The Cost of Complexity

The complexity of the American multi-payer health care system staggers the mind. I have drawn the diagram shown in the top portion of Figure 6.1 in an attempt to depict graphically the various flows of billing and payments through the system. The diagram is strikingly complex because of the highly fragmented nature of our health care system. The diagram, undoubtedly incomplete, suggests more than twenty money-flow paths and more than thirty billing paths between the consuming public and the health care providers and drug suppliers. (Compare the top portion of Figure 6.1 with the bottom portion, showing the flows in the United Kingdom's unified and very simple health care system, to be discussed in Chapter 7.)

Another important feature of the top portion of Figure 6.1, one easy to miss, is its depiction of the central role that private insurance companies play in the American health care system. Sitting there in the center of the diagram, the private insurance

UNITED STATES' MULTI-PAYER HEALTH CARE SYSTEM

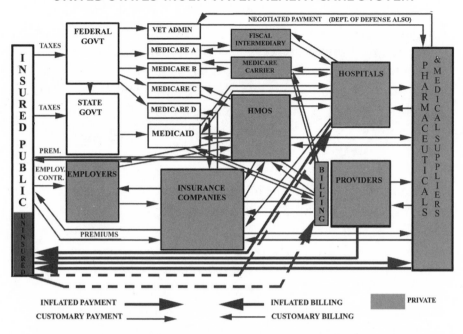

| INFLATED PAYMENT | ➡ | ⬅ | INFLATED BILLING | PRIVATE |
| CUSTOMARY PAYMENT | → | ← | CUSTOMARY BILLING | |

UNITED KINGDOM'S UNIVERSAL HEALTH CARE SYSTEM

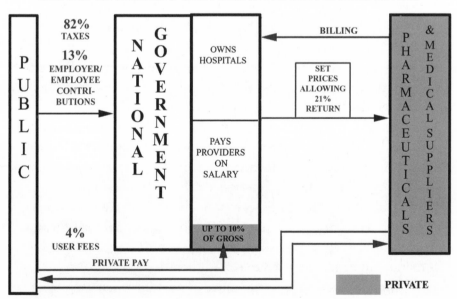

Figure 6.1 - Diagrams depicting the flow of billings and payments in the American health care system, at top, and at bottom that in the United Kingdom's much simpler system. Arrows pointing to the left indicate billings, and those pointing to the right indicate payments. See also Figures 7.1 to 7.3 to be presented later, pp. 122–133.

companies—in their roles as fiscal intermediaries, Medicare carriers, and policy insurers—control a major portion of the dollar flow between American citizens and their medical and drug providers. In the process they absorb roughly 20 to 30 percent of the money the United States spends on its health care. That money goes to substantial shareholder profits and large administrative costs.

In discussing the American or any other health care system, we need to keep in mind one important fact: health care spending roughly follows the 80/20 rule noted earlier (20 percent of the population will account for 80 percent of expenses.) Similarly, half of the population has virtually no medical expenses, whereas 1 percent accounts for 22 percent of expenses.[97] The unavoidable consequence of this fact is that a responsible society must devise some equitable way to spread the burden of health care costs over a much broader segment of the society than solely the one incurring the bulk of the expenses. That smaller segment simply is not capable of paying for the costs it incurs.

The most common method modern governments use to cover health care costs is to collect money from their citizens and then either provide the health care themselves, as in the United Kingdom, or, as in Canada, directly pay independent hospitals and providers for the necessary services without regard to which elements of the society require the services. In certain of these universal health care systems, some people using the services may be required, only if financially able, to co-pay a small portion of the costs, but a major fraction of the cost of health care is borne directly by the government. Such systems are sometimes described as having government-provided "universal health care insurance," but it needs to be understood that "insurance" really is merely a mechanism used to pay for health care.

That distinction becomes more important when we look at the American health care system because of the several kinds of insurance it uses—along with direct user-to-provider payments—to reimburse hospitals and other health care providers. Through its Veterans Administration the government directly provides health care to veterans. Long vilified due to past failings, this strictly socialistic system has so reformed itself in recent years that is now considered to be the country's best healthcare system.[98, †] The VA system has managed this remarkable feat while holding costs well below those of the other portions of the overall national healthcare system, and it covers the full cost of care—no co-pays, deductibles or coverage caps.

Better known to the general public are two government "insurance" programs that serve special segments of the population: Medicare that serves the elderly, and Medicaid that serves those financially unable to pay for medical care regardless of their age. Unlike the fully socialistic VA healthcare program, these systems are socialistic only to the extent that the insurance is government provided; the private sector provides the health care. The Medicaid program seeks to cover the full cost of health care required by users, whereas the Medicare program pays only the major portion, roughly 80 percent, and requires users to pay the rest, either directly or by purchasing **supplemental medical insurance** from the private sector.

As Table 6.3 shows, the federal and state governments pick up well over one-third of the direct costs of health care through the several programs, leaving the public and its employers to pay for the rest, roughly 60 percent. The bulk of that other money is funneled through for-profit private insurance companies; however, some 47 million or more Americans do not have insurance and so they pay directly to providers on a fee-for–service basis for whatever health care they receive—to the extent that they are financially able. Others pay for health care by a combination of direct pay and purchasing of health insurance, and employers pay for a significant portion of the insurance.

Unique to America, employer-provided insurance, which began as a consequence of labor shortages during World War II, has, as noted earlier, become a major element in healthcare

---

† Note that military hospitals such as Walter Reed and Tripler, which have recently received much criticism in the press, are not VA hospitals—they are army hospitals.

finance. However, it is now undergoing retrenchment as employers face increasing insurance costs and competition overseas from companies in countries having less expensive healthcare systems and less employer responsibility in paying for health care. Employers are divesting themselves of both cost and risk by requiring employees to pay higher co-pays and increased contributions for insurance coverage. They also are seeking to lower costs by screening out potential employees with health problems.

Americans with healthcare insurance are under attack from another front as well: the for-profit private insurance companies. By refusing payment for some medical services and by identifying high-cost customers and raising their policy rates or rejecting them outright, these companies are simultaneously reducing payouts and raising profits.[99]

The consequences of these employer and insurance company trends are severe. By effectively forcing higher co-payment for medical services, they put increasing numbers of people in the position of having to expend higher portions of their income on health care and they are forcing more people into the ranks of the uninsured. Uninsured people suffer from poorer health than insured persons and they die sooner. The National Academies' Institute of Medicine estimates that 18,000 people die prematurely each year as a result of being uninsured.[100]

The uninsured segment of the public pays what it can directly for its health care, often at rates higher than the insured, and for a lower level of health care than the fully insured public. Some cannot afford to pay more than a portion of the cost of their health care, and so our system shifts a portion of the cost of serving the uninsured sector over to the insured sector, and the insured sector also picks up whatever costs the Medicare and Medicaid programs may fail to provide for the clientele they serve.

Except for the very rich, every member of the American public suffers from the deficiencies in our healthcare system. Its fragmentation creates abnormally high administrative costs—said to be approximately 30 percent—that are mostly unnecessary, as is readily seen when we go on to examine the healthcare systems of other countries.

It is not just the consuming public that suffers from the fragmentation; the members of the medical profession have to endure the hardships as well. Those medical providers not directly employed by government agencies face a prodigious task just to get paid for their services, whether their patients are covered by Medicare, Medicaid, other insurance, or no insurance at all. The providers are forced into hiring staff to fill out multitudinous billing forms and to spend an undue amount of their own time on paperwork, time they would much prefer to spend doing what they were trained for: to provide health care to patients.

Every healthcare system has its deficiencies, but the American system takes the cake, and is rightly described as dysfunctional. It is terribly expensive, and getting more so by the year, yet it fails to provide the health care that the citizens of a modern nation should have.

The New International Health Tourism Industry

Interestingly enough, the high cost of medical care in the United States combined with the lack of health insurance for approximately 47 million Americans is now creating increasing traffic overseas to Asia and elsewhere for medical care.[‡] High-quality medical care is becoming increasingly available in such countries as Thailand and India that are actively pursuing development of medical centers. Some with American certification are attracting foreigners because of the high quality and low cost of health care they provide. Uninsured Americans, in particular, are attracted because costs in these centers can be as low as one-tenth that in the United States, and travel costs in comparison can pale to insignificance. Contributing to this so-called health tourism industry are some American insurance companies who

---

[‡] I am told that some Alaskans go to Whitehorse, Yukon Territory, Canada, for dental care.

find it cheaper to outsource their covered patients to these new centers rather than pay for their care in the United States. In India, a heart-valve replacement procedure costing $200,000 in the U.S. is about $10,000, including round-trip airfare and a brief vacation package.[101]

Increasingly famous is the luxurious Brumrungrad Hospital in Bangkok, where open-heart surgery costs about $7,000 and hospital beds $50 per night. State-of-the-art, this hospital claims to serve more foreigners than any other in the world, and in 2004 some 60,000 Americans used its services for such procedures as hip and knee replacements, open-heart surgery, dental work, and cosmetic surgery.[102] The very poorest Americans are less able to take advantage of the international healthcare market, but those who can are likely to put increasing pressure on the American healthcare system to lower its costs.

53. U.S. Department of Commerce, Bureau of Economic Analysis; www.bea.gov/newsreleases/glance.htm.

54. Office of Management and Budget; www.whitehouse.gov/omb/budget/fy2002/guide02.html.

55. The MetLife market survey of nursing home & home care costs, April 2002 and September 2005, MetLife Mature Market Institute; www.lifeplansinc.com.

56. Centers for Medicare & Medicaid Services; www.cms.hhs.gov/NationalHealthExpendData/.

57. Conan, Cathy A., and Micah B. Hartman, Financing health care: businesses, households, and governments, 1987-2003, *Health Care Financing Review*/Web Exclusive/July 2005.

58. 2002–2003 State Health Expenditure Report, Co-Published by the Milbank Memorial Fund, the National Association of State Budget Officers, and the Reforming States Group; www.milbank.org/reports/2000scher/.

59. Friedman, Milton, How to cure health care, *Hoover Digest*, 2001, No. 3; www.hooverdigest.org/013/friedman.html, and Sereo, Susan Starr, and Rushika Fernandopulle, *Uninsured in America: Life and death in the land of opportunity* (Berkeley: University of California Press, 2005) p. 192.

60. California Medical Association, How to compare health plans; www.cmanet.org/PUBLICDOC.cfm/57/5.

61. Health Insurance Info; www.healthinsurance.info/plans/Traditional-Health-Insurance.HTM.

62. America's Health Insurance Plans; www.ahip.org/content/default.aspx?bc=31|42.

63. Pear, Robert, Loss of competition is seen in health insurance industry, *The New York Times*, April 30, 2006; www.nytimes.com/2006/04/30/us/30insure. html?ex=1189137600&en=e86c154e54782b0d&ei=5070.

64. Palmetto GBA, 2006 Annual report; www.palmettogba.com/palmetto/ aboutarea.nsf/pdf/2006_annual_report.pdf.

65. Wikipedia, Blue Cross and Blue Shield Association; http://en.wikipedia.org/ wiki/Blue_Cross_and_Blue_Shield_Association#_note-0.

66. BlueCross BlueShield Association, History of Blue Cross Shield; www.bcbs. com/about/history/.

67. BlueCross BlueShield Association, Covering America; www.bcbs.com/about/ history/covering-america.html.

68. WellPoint, Inc. 2006 Summary Annual Report; http://media.corporate-ir.net/ media_files/irol/13/130104/reports/wlp_2006_AR_v2.pdf.

69. Friedman, Mark, For-profit health insurance carriers getting the blues, *Arkansas Business*, May 22, 2006; www.arkansasbusiness.com/article.aspx?aID=94379.945 10.106523.

70. S. Woolhandler and D.U. Himmelstein, *The National Health Program Slide-show Guide*, 2000, quoted by John P. Geyman, *International Journal of Health Services*, Vol. 35, No. 1, 2005.

71. Woolhandler, S., et al. Costs of health care administration in the United States and Canada, *New England J. Medicine*, 768-775, 2003.

72. National Coalition on Health Care, Facts on health care costs; www.nchc.org/ facts/2007%20updates/cost.pdf.

73. National Coalition on Health Care, Health insurance cost; www.nchc.org/ facts/cost.shtml.

74. Friedman, Mark, For-profit health insurance carriers getting the blues, *Arkansas Business*, May 22, 2006; www.arkansasbusiness.com/article.aspx?aID=94379.945 10.106523.

75. *The New York Times*, Associated Press, Humana earnings soar in quarter, July 31, 2007; www.nytimes.com/2007/07/31/business/31humana.html?ex=118939680 0&en=76e5db4f3a97088f&ei=5070.

76. Mattera, Phil, Private health insurance is not the answer, AlterNet, February 23, 2007; www.alternet.org/story/48371/.

77. National Center For Policy Analysis, Risk pools: a better solution, June 30, 1994; www.ncpa.org/ba/ba112.html.

78. OneCareNOW.org, Multiple health insurance risk pools fail to control costs; www.onecarenow.org/healthcarereformriskpools.htm.

79. Alaska Department of Health & Social Services, data presented at Fairbanks regional forum on health care coverage, July 24, 2007.

80. U.S. Census Bureau, GCT-T1, Population Estimates, 2006; http://factfinder. census.gov/servlet/GCTTable?_bm=y&-geo_id=01000US&-_box_head_ nbr=GCT-T1&-ds_name=PEP_2006_EST&-_lang=en&-format=US-9&-_sse=on.

81. Graham, Judith, 'Underinsured' skimping on health care, study says, *Chicago Tribune*, June 14, 2005; www.chicagotribune.com/features/lifestyle/health/chi-060103insurance2-story,1,4544168.story.

82. The Commonwealth Fund, Gaps in health insurance: an all-American problem, April 26, 2006; www.commonwealthfund.org/publications/publications_show. htm?doc_id=367876.

83. Foster, Mark, and Scott Goldsmith, Alaska's $5 billion health care bill—who's paying, UA Research Summary No. 6, Institute of Social and Economic Research, University of Alaska Anchorage, March 2006.

84. Indian health Service, Facts on Indian health disparities, January 2007; http:// info.ihs.gov/Files/DisparitiesFacts-Jan2007.doc.

85. Alaska Department of Health & Social Services, data presented at Fairbanks regional forum on health care coverage, July 24, 2007.

86. Sered, Susan Starr, and Rushika Fernandopule, *Uninsured in America: Life and death in the land of opportunity*, University of California Press, Berkeley, 2005, p. 1 and following.

87. Ibid., p. 13.

88. Alaska Department of Revenue, Permanent Fund Division; https://www.pfd. state.ak.us/.

89. Alaska Permanent Fund Corporation; www.apfc.org/.

90. Banner Health, Financial assistance programs; www.bannerhealth.com/_ Patients+and+Visitors/Financial+Assistance+Programs.htm.

91. Employee Benefit Management Services, Inc (EBMS), Claims cost containment; www.ebmstpa.com/Default.aspx?cID=29.

92. Based on my examination of billing and payment statements.

93. Medicare 2005 Handbook; www.merritt-gentry.com/freefiles/files/ MEDICARE.HTM.

94. The Henry J. Kaiser Family Foundation Fact Sheet: Medicare at a glance, September 2005; www.kff.org.

95. Tufts Managed Care Institute, A brief history of managed care, 1998; www.tmci. org/downloads/BriefHist.pdf.

96. Kazel, Robert, Are HMOs dead? *American Medical News*, April 18, 2005; www. ama-assn.org/amednews/2005/04/18/bisa0418.htm.

97. Krugman, Paul, and Robin Williams, The health care crisis and what to do about it, *The New York Review of Books*, Vol. 53, No. 5, March 23, 2006; www. nybooks.com/articles/18802.

98. Longman, Phillip, The best care anywhere, *Washington Monthly*, January/ February 2005; www.washingtonmonthly.com/features/2005/0501.longman. html.

99. Snowbeck, Christopher, Health insurer profits triple, *Pittsburgh Post-Gazette*, March 24, 2005; www.post-gazette.com/pg/05083/476795.stm.

100. Banibeau, Simone, Health insurance crisis worsens while Aetna posts profits, *The New Standard*, May 1, 2004; http://newstandardnews.net/content/index. cfm/items/268.

101. *UDaily*, University of Delaware, Medical tourism grows worldwide; www.udel. edu/PR/UDaily/2005/mar/tourism072505.html.

102. Mydans, Seth, The perfect Thai vacation: sun, sea and surgery, *The New York Times: International,* September 9, 2002; www.fieldworking.com/main/ schoolHouse/engagingThai.html#OG.

7

*Americans are clueless on what
happens in other countries.*

—ROBERT H. LEBOW, M.D.

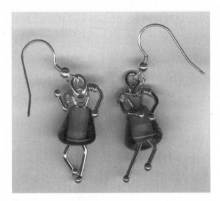

Comparison of Our System with that of Canada and Other Countries

must admit that, prior to the experience with Patricia, I had given only cursory thought to the American health care system in general, and even less to that of other nations. Although I had spent time in other countries, my contacts with their health care systems were minimal, highly satisfactory, and cost-free. After receiving an eye injury while participating in a rocket launching expedition off the coast of Peru, I went into an immaculate clinic in Lima where the doctor saw me shortly after I walked in the door, patched me up, and, while shrugging his shoulders, used both hands to wave me away when I tried to pay. The same thing happened in Toronto, Canada, when on a visit there my wife Rosemarie seemed to be coming down with something. We went to a local clinic where she was taken in immediately, examined and given some pills. When we asked the receptionist how much we owed, she got a blank look on her face and replied, "I don't know, why don't you forget about it, eh?" Events like these don't happen in America, the land of the bold and the free. Obviously, things are different "overseas."

The comparison and evaluation of national health care systems is not an easy matter. The financial cost of a system is a significant factor, but equally important is how well a system maintains the health of its people. In 2000 the World Health Organization published a report on the health care systems of its 191 member countries, rating them according to several broadly stated measures.[103] The measures included the overall level of health in each country, how well the health care is distributed, the level and distribution of system responsiveness, fairness in financial contribution, how well the system meets expectations, and the expenditure per capita. The study makes use of specific objective indicators of system effectiveness such as the longevity of the citizenry and infant mortality rates, and also more subjective measures relating to the use of available resources and the fairness of their application. All of these are then combined to rate overall system performance. The United States' health care system does not come out well in this scheme: its overall system performance ranks in 37th place, below the ratings of all other fully industrialized nations. One consolation, however, is that we handily beat out Russia and China, rated 130th and 144th, respectively.

Characteristics of National Health Care Systems

Among the world's industrialized nations, the United States has the most expensive health system per capita, and the only one that does not seek to provide all citizens with basic health care services. As one source puts it, "Some form of social medical insurance exists in every European and Pacific Rim nation as well as Canada, Australia and New Zealand. In fact, the United States is the only nation in both NATO and the twenty-four nation Organization for Economic Cooperation and Development (OECD) that does not extend medical coverage to all of its citizens."[104]

The health care systems in these countries all differ from one another, blending in varying degrees of **capitalism** and **socialism**. However, they all are predicated on the view that health care, like education, is a human right that the government has a responsibility to provide—and they are all cheaper to run than the American system which does not operate on the same premise. In America, health care is a privilege, not a right.

In discussing various national health care systems, it is important to distinguish what is meant by the terminology used, especially so because of some of the mythology surrounding the discussion and the use of certain evocative or provocative words in propaganda tracts intended to glorify the American system. Among the most used are 'social,' 'socialism,' and 'socialize.' These three words sound pretty much the same, but the latter two have quite different meaning from the first. 'Social' has several meanings all related to interactions between individuals, togetherness, and communal activities. By contrast, 'socialism' and 'socialize' have specific meaning related directly to ownership. Webster defines socialism as "any of various theories or systems of ownership and operation of the means of production and distribution by society or the community rather than by private individuals, with all members of society or the community sharing in the work and the products." Similarly, Webster gives the relevant definition of 'socialize' as meaning "to subject to governmental ownership and control; nationalize." The key word in both of these latter definitions is 'ownership,' and that is important to remember when discussing health care systems. A socialized system is one involving actual government ownership of the system, as contrasted to a capitalistic system, in which the ownership is private.

In the United Kingdom the government owns the hospitals and clinics, and it directly employs physicians and other health care personnel to operate them. Thus the term **socialized medicine** rightly describes the British health care system. Canada, on the other hand, does not have socialized medicine. Instead, it has a single-payer health care system not involving government ownership of facilities or direct employment of health care personnel. The government regulates health care and collects and distributes money to pay for it. Ninety-five percent of Canadian hospitals are privately owned nonprofits.[105] Therefore, it definitely is a misuse of terminology to describe the Canadian system as socialistic; it is a strictly capitalistic system. Actually, the American health care system involves more socialism than the Canadian because the American government owns the Veterans Administration and other hospitals and it directly hires medical personnel to operate them. An essential distinction is that the United States has a multi-payer system that does not provide health care to all citizens, whereas Canada and the United Kingdom have single-payer universal health care systems that provide health care for all.

Unfortunately, Americans have so often been told that Canada has socialized medicine that many believe it. Worse yet, the term socialized medicine has evolved from its actual meaning to one used, especially by propagandists and right-wing politicians, to describe any health care system controlled and financed by government. An extreme example is contained in a speech by Republican presidential candidate Rudy Giuliani in July 2007. He said:

> We've got to do it the American way. The American way is not single-payer, government-controlled anything. That's a European way of doing something; that's frankly a socialist way of doing something. That's why when you hear Democrats in particular talk about single-mandated health care, universal health care, what they're talking about is socialized medicine.[106]

Such associations of universal health care with socialized medicine are unfortunate, as they tend to create a negative anti-socialism knee-jerk reaction in many Americans that inhibits rational discussion of universal health care.

Most of the nations with universal health care systems have had them in operation for several decades, but Taiwan is an example of a nation that recently joined the group. Before 1995, Taiwan had a multiple insurance company payment system like that of the United States. It then instituted a national single-payer coverage program, and found that the change did not incur any increase in costs. The cost of bringing 8 million uninsured citizens (out of a total population of 22 million) into the system was easily covered by the savings from operating the single-payer system.[107]

With the exception of the Canadian system, we in the United States do not hear much about the health care systems of other countries, and so we know little about them. In his recent book *Health Care Meltdown*,[108] physician Robert H. LeBow puts it more strongly: "Americans are clueless on what happens in other countries." It is actually worse than that when it comes to knowing about the Canadian health care system, because special-interest groups have subjected Americans to misinformation campaigns seeking to downplay the Canadian system's advantages while stressing the disadvantages. In the 1990s, the American Medical Association launched a major campaign toward that end, and in 2000 the pharmaceutical industry spent an estimated $60 million on an ad campaign to discredit the Canadian system.[109]

The Canadian Health Care System

The Canadian health care system (called medicare) does have its problems, mostly traceable to underfunding enforced by conservative political interests during recent years. Whereas the United States spends 16 percent of its Gross Domestic Product on health care, Canada has been spending far less, about 10 percent. Although the majority of Canadians are highly satisfied with their system, they are now embroiled in much discussion, and conservative elements of Canadian society are promoting change that would make it more administratively dependent on commercial enterprise, as in the United States.[110]

The foundation of the current health care system in Canada is the Canadian Health Care Act of 1984 that defines the system and lays out the principles on which it operates. The act makes the ten Canadian provincial and three territorial governments the key providers of health care and requires them to operate under certain federal guidelines. They are required to make basic health care available to every citizen, but are allowed some freedom as to how that is to be provided, subject to five guiding principles:

1—Health care must be universal; that is, available to all citizens.

2—Health care must be portable. Every citizen must be able to obtain health care in every province, by whatever hospital or other provider the citizen chooses.

3—Health care must be comprehensive. It must provide fully for health care deemed medically necessary (nose-bobs and facelifts don't count).

4—Health care must be accessible. All citizens must have access.

5—Health care must be publicly administered—for-profit commercial enterprises cannot participate in its administration.

The federal government enforces these principles by its power to withhold funding from regional governments that fail to conform, although the provinces and territories provide the major share of funding through taxation or other means such as requiring health insurance premiums, as do Alberta and British Columbia.

The provincially funded healthcare system covers only medical care that is considered essential, and generally does not cover dental and hearing care, or such services as in-vitro fertilization (rules vary from province to province). These other services are either out-of-pocket expenses or covered by private insurance, as in the United States.

One major difference between the Canadian and American systems is the payment system for hospital care. Canadian hospitals are mostly privately owned, not-for-profit institutions, and they do not bill for individual patient services. Instead, they receive from the provinces annual global payments that are negotiated between the provinces and the hospitals. The simplicity of this system allows low hospital administrative cost, about one-half the roughly 20-percent administrative cost of operating American hospitals.

Most of the payment to physicians and other nonhospital providers is more akin to the American system in that these healthcare providers are mostly private and are paid on a fee-for-service basis through billings to the provincial governments. The billings for these services must be in the amounts specified in a negotiated "Schedule of Benefits," each province having its own schedule. Thus the inequities created by arbitrarily high 'actual billing' in the United States disappear in Canada. The fee-for-service payment schedules in Canada differ from those based on the American system by tending to use more descriptive terms than the numerical designations embodied in the HCPCS coding system used in the United States. Nevertheless, a download of one of the provincial payment schedules creates a several-hundred-page document, so the Canadian schedule of payments to nonhospital providers appears on the surface to be comparable in complexity. However, statistical data indicate that the human effort and administrative cost for nonhospital Canadian health care providers is about half that of American providers. The relative simplicity of the system is indicated in the diagram in Figure 7.1. Compare with Figure 6.1, presented earlier (p. 107).

Canadian physicians can opt out of the national medicare system, but if they do they are not allowed to receive any public monies, and they are not allowed to charge more for services than

CANADA'S UNIVERSAL HEALTH CARE SYSTEM

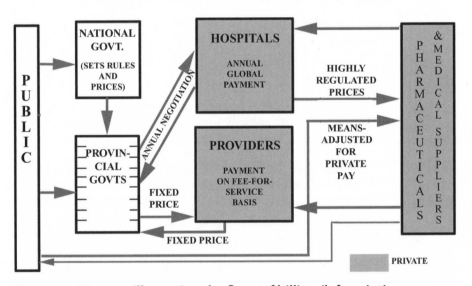

Figure 7.1 Diagram illustrating the flows of billing (left-pointing arrows) and payments (right-pointing arrows) in the Canadian health care system. The system cost is 43 percent of that of the American system, and the World Health Organization rates it higher in overall effectiveness: in 30th place versus 37th place for the United States. Compare with Figure 6.1, p. 107.

is allowed by the Schedule of Benefits. That requirement coupled with a provision of the Canada Health Care Act specifically prohibiting a Canadian citizen from buying from the private sector any service covered by the public health system means that an opted-out physician can deliver to Canadians only the noncore services not covered by the Canadian medicare system. However, he could provide the core services listed in the Schedule of Benefits to noncitizens, but only at the rates specified by the schedule. These rates are likely to be lower than the "customary, prevailing, or reasonable" rates American health care providers are paid by Medicare or insurance companies, so the situation is conducive to a flow of Americans across the border simply to get cheaper medical care or to undergo procedures available in Canada but not in the United States. Some American health insurance plans do allow payment to private Canadian health care providers.

Costs of the Canadian and American Health Care Systems

Table 7.1 presents data on the per capita cost of various components of health care in Canada and the United States. The table illustrates two major points:

> ▶ 1. Spending for health care is radically different in the two countries. In 1999 the United States spent $4,359 per capita while Canada was spending only $2,463, 57 percent of the United States amount.

> ▶ 2. Administrative cost of the health care system in the United States was twice that of the Canadian system, 24 percent versus 12 percent of the money spent for health care in the nation.

These are startling facts, considered that by every major measure used to evaluate health care—such things as infant

Table 7.1 - Cost of administering health care in Canada and the United States in 1999. Based on a table by S. Woolhandler et al.[111] as quoted by John P. Geyman.[112]

Cost Category	Spending per Capita, in United States Dollars		Ratio US/Canada
	United States	Canada	
Insurance Overhead	$259	$47	5.5
Employers' Costs	$57	$8	7.1
Hospital Administration	$315	$103	3.1
Nursing Home Administration	$62	$29	2.1
Practitioners' Administration	$324	$107	3.0
Home Care Administration	$42	$13	3.2
Total Administration Cost	$1,059	$307	3.4
Total Health Care Spending[113]	$4,358	$2,463	1.73
Percent Administration Cost	24%	12%	2.0

mortality rates, longevity, and fairness—Canada rates higher than the United States. The United States is perhaps spending too much money on health care, and it definitely is putting way too much money into the wrong places—namely into administration and corporate profit.

A telling commentary about the difference between costs of the American and Canadian healthcare systems—and also the large cut taken from the health care dollar by corporate profits and administrative costs—was voiced some years ago by two authorities from the Harvard Medical School, David U. Himmelstein and Steffie Woolhandler.[114] They pointed out that the profit and overhead taken by large American managed healthcare organizations (HMOs) is about 30 percent, and that private insurers in the States take about 13 percent of premium dollars for profit and overhead. Yet the American Medicare program direct overhead consumes less that 2 percent, and the Canadian medicare program less than 1 percent. So much for the argument that private enterprise is always more efficient than government, and, therefore, privatization is always better.

These authors also note that in the 1990s Blue Cross in Massachusetts employed more people to administer healthcare coverage of 2.5 million New Englanders than were employed in all of Canada to administer single-payer coverage for 27 million Canadians. And as shown in Table 7.1, Canadian hospitals spend only about one-third as much for administration as do American hospitals. In Massachusetts, hospitals were spending about 25 percent of their revenues on billing and administration. Similarly, Canadian physicians require less than half the clerical and managerial staff of their American counterparts.

It is evident that Canada's single-payer system and method of global payment to hospitals allows a level of efficiency impossible to reach with America's system of multiple payers and its hospital billing on a per-patient basis. The multiple payer system imposes a heavy bureaucratic burden on hospitals because they must bill several insurance programs, each having different and sometimes voluminous regulations on coverage, and of course the same is true of nonhospital medical providers in the United States.

Quite obviously, say Himmelstein and Woolhandler, the United States needs to establish a single-payer healthcare system, one that provides health care to all its citizens.

The Much-touted Canadian Wait List 'Problem'

The main thing Americans hear about the Canadian system is the problem of long wait times, weeks and even months for non-emergency procedures. This issue is a much-discussed topic among critics of Canadian medicare on both sides of the border, and opponents of a single-payer system (such as the American health insurance industry) tout this and the related issue of healthcare rationing as major arguments against the system.

While there can be no question that long wait lists do exist for certain procedures, it appears that reliable statistics are mostly lacking, in part because of nonuniform definitions of what determines when a person is considered to be on a wait list. Also there appears to be much variation with location. For example, one source[115] states that waiting times for CT scans in Manitoba range from 3 to 18 weeks, depending upon the location of the hospital.

Waiting times also vary much with procedure, mainly because of differences in availability of personnel. This same source notes that in British Columbia the median waiting time for vascular surgery was 2.7 weeks, while that for gall bladder surgery was 5.1 weeks, orthopedic surgery 9.3 weeks, hip replacement 21.8 weeks, and knee replacement 28.3 weeks.

The numbers seem to depend upon who is giving them, and a few sources cite, usually anecdotally, very long waits of over a year in some cases. What appears to be unbiased information comes from Statistics Canada,[116] a nonpartisan organization. Reporting government data, it states that in 2003 the median waiting time for elective surgery in Canada was 4.3 weeks; wait time to see a specialist for a new illness, 4.0 weeks; and for non-emergency diagnostic testing, 3.0 weeks. This source states that in 2003 to 2005 median wait times for all specialized services were 3 to 4 weeks, and that 70 to 80 percent of Canadian patients deemed these wait times as acceptable.

At first glance it would appear that one solution to the wait list problem is to put more money into the system. Another proposed solution is to allow those Canadians who can afford it to buy services from the private sector, thereby setting up a two-tier system more akin to the American healthcare system. Opinions in Canada are much divided on this idea. There is fear that setting up a two-tier system would not solve the problem, and that it would damage the current single-payer system. One group of Canadian physicians[117] argues against both of the two above options and suggests instead that the wait list problem could be reduced simply by better management procedures made increasingly feasible by modern communication and information processing capabilities. Their specific suggestions include coordination of wait lists so that referrals could be made to clinicians with shorter wait lists, more careful auditing of wait lists to reorder them according to patient need and to reduce backlogging caused by missed appointments (apparently more than a minor problem), and also trying to reduce the number of followup visits by busy specialists.

It so happens that as I write this I am waiting in Alaska for an appointment with a physician that is set for 5 weeks from the time of the first request, and also for a non-emergency diagnostic test coming 10 weeks from first contact with the physician doing the testing. Wait times such as these are common here in interior Alaska, and perhaps elsewhere in the United States. The point is that wait times for non-emergency medical services do not automatically drop to zero when a person crosses Canada's southern and western borders. For the uninsured person in the U.S., waits for medical service can be measured in lifetimes rather than weeks. Obviously, rationing of medical services takes place in both Canada and the United States. The Canadians do it on the basis of availability of services, and the Americans do it on the basis of ability to pay. Which way is best might be debatable, but longevity and other healthcare statistics make it hard to argue for the superiority of the American method of rationing healthcare services.

Related to the wait list problem in Canada is what we hear about Canadians crossing the border to the United States for health care. This matter also is touted as a telling argument against the Canadian system; however, it appears that the argument may have little basis in fact. Rather interesting results come from a recent study described by a group of American and Canadian authors.[118] They offer five possible reasons why Canadians might seek health care in the United States: 1—Services are available in Canada but involve long wait times, 2—Leading-edge technologies might be unavailable in Canada, 3—Rural residents living near the border find it easier to cross than to travel to Canadian health centers, 4—Snowbirds (Canadians staying in the United States during the colder months) or business and leisure travelers use locally available services rather than to return home for health care, and 5—The perception that certain American health centers (such as the Mayo clinics in Minnesota, Florida and Arizona) might offer better services.

Some results from the study:

▶ Of 18,000 Canadians responding to a 1996 survey, 90 had received health care in the United States, and only 20 had gone there specifically for health care.

▶ As a result of Canadian provinces contracting with nearby U.S. hospitals, 8.5 percent of Canadians undergoing radiation therapy for prostate and breast cancer received that treatment in the United States.

▶ Quebec approves about 100 requests per year for treatments in U.S. hospitals that are unavailable in that province.

▶ From 1994 to 1998, 2,031 Canadians were admitted to hospitals in Michigan, 1,689 to hospitals in New York, and 825 to hospitals in Washington. These U.S. hospitalizations were 0.23 percent of the total hospitalizations in the three bordering provinces.

The authors of this study concluded that relatively few Canadians crossed the border for medical services, and that in many cases the reasons were less related to long Canadian wait times than to other circumstances such as emergency care coincident with travel to the United States. Another cause was provincial contracting with near-border American hospitals and clinics for services in short supply at home, benefiting both the Canadian patients and American facilities having excess capacity. The overall conclusion was that the claims of major southward border crossings for medical care were based more on myth than reality. They state:

Despite the evidence presented in our study, the Canadian border-crossing claims will probably persist. The tension between payers and providers is real, inevitable, and permanent, and claims that serve the interests of either party will continue to be independent of the evidentiary base. Debates over health policy furnish a number of examples of these 'zombies'—ideas that, on logic or evidence, are intellectually dead—that can never be laid to rest because they are useful to some powerful interests. The phantom hordes of Canadian refugees are likely to remain among them.

Minor northbound traffic across the U.S.-Canada border for health care also exists because some Americans have crossed over to undergo procedures offered in Canada but not yet approved in the United States, and of course there has been considerable traffic involving the purchasing of pharmaceuticals in Canada by Americans. Another form of medical traffic results from the fact that in Canada the education of doctors and nurses is essentially free, but costly in the United States. Although both nurses and doctors are in short supply in Canada, some of them have moved to the United States because wages in certain specialties are higher there. (In the 1990s some 300 of 50,000 Canadian doctors were moving to the United States each year.) Recently in the news were stories about American near-border hospitals having difficulties because many of their nurses were Canadian residents who were having trouble crossing the border to work because of new regulations being imposed by American Homeland Security.

It is important to remember that the discussions of wait times that we hear usually refer only to elective procedures. In both countries we see in the literature anecdotal horror stories telling about people in critical conditions failing to get timely emergency room care, but statistical information indicates that emergency room wait times are roughly about the same in Canada and the United States.[119] According to examinations of wait times by the governments involved, 96 percent of ER patients in the United Kingdom spend less than four hours in emergency rooms (from the time they arrive, are treated, and then released), 76 percent of Canadians spend less than that, but only 72 percent of American patients spend less than four hours. In Canada the median wait time for a patient with serious need to see a physician quickly is about five minutes.[120]

Other National Health Care Systems

Following the lead of Ezra Klein, a writer and co-editor of www.pandagon.net, an Internet journal of political and cultural commentary, I now briefly summarize the health care systems of four other countries: France, Germany, Japan, and the United Kingdom.[121] Like Canada—and, let me remind you, like all other modern nations except the United States—these countries have universal health care systems that are less expensive and rate higher in effectiveness than the American system. Many smaller countries, also all with universal health care systems, rate higher than the United States according to the *World Health Organization Annual Report (2000)*.[122] Among them are Australia, Austria, Belgium, Italy, Norway, Spain, Sweden, and The Netherlands.

France

Rated by the World Health Organization (WHO) as having the best health care system of its 191 member states, the French system covers every citizen with insurance. Its reimbursement rates are wholly uniform. (No inflated actual billings allowed.) Seventy-five percent of the funding is public (collected by income tax) with the remainder coming from employer and employee contributions. The money is funneled into three non-competing funds jointly controlled by employers and unions, and is supervised by the state. France is the only major country with unlimited access to health care: patients can go to specialists and nonspecialists alike, although the system is now being changed to require nonspecialist referrals to specialists. The state operates hospitals and allocates to them specialized equipment, but also allows private hospitals that operate on a regulated fee-for-service basis. French physicians make far less than their American counterparts but receive essentially free medical training. Figure 7.2 depicts the flow of money and billings through this system.

FRANCE'S UNIVERSAL HEALTH CARE SYSTEM

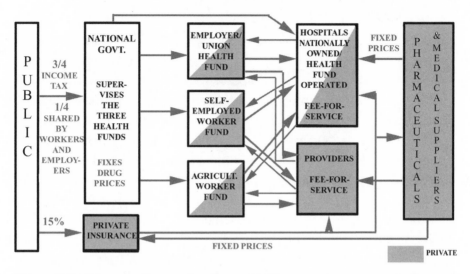

Figure 7.2 - Diagram illustrating flow of billings and payments in France's health care system, billings flowing to the left, payments to the right. The cost of the French system is 57 percent that of the American system. The World Health Organization rates France's system in first place among its 191 member nations.

Compare with similar diagrams for the United States (Figure 6.1 top portion, p. 107), Canada (Figure 7.1, p. 122), and the United Kingdom (Figure 7.3, p. 133).

Japan

Rated by WHO in tenth place, Japan has a universal health care system that is about 75 percent publicly funded through payroll taxes. It has three components. One involves about 26 percent of the population that is covered by payroll-tax-funded employer-managed plans required of all employers having 700+ employees and which the employers manage. Employees and dependents of smaller employers (about 30 percent of the population) are covered by a government-operated health plan. These two components are required to contribute to about 40 percent of the cost of a third plan that covers retirees and all other citizens, including their long-term care when required. The remainder of that cost comes from general revenue. All three plans cover a wide range of benefits that include dental care, maternity care, and prescription drugs. All privately owned hospitals and clinics (about 80 percent of the total) are nonprofit. The government operates all large hospitals but there are many small hospitals and clinics that are family-owned and operated by independent doctors. All hospitals and clinics operate on a fee-for-service basis with the fees fixed by the government, as are prescription drug prices. Co-pays of 10 percent to 20 percent are required, but are lower for those of limited income, and the elderly do not co-pay for prescriptions. Japan's physicians in public and private hospitals are salaried.[123]

United Kingdom

Rated in 18th place by WHO, the United Kingdom has a universal healthcare system that serves every resident as well as overseas students, refugees and asylum seekers. It is funded 82 percent through general taxes, 13 percent from employer and employee contributions, and 4 percent from user fees. The system requires each person to choose any general practitioner he wants as his primary care physician. This physician then acts as a **gatekeeper** for access to specialists who typically work in hospitals and receive a salary from the National Health Service, which also operates hospitals. The general practitioners are under contract with the health service and are paid on a per-patient (**capitation**) basis but are also allowed to simultaneously treat private-pay patients on a regulated fee-for-service basis. The hospital-based specialists are allowed to earn up to 10 percent of their gross pay by treating private-pay patients. In addition to physicians, important healthcare providers are midwives who are registered nurses having further qualifications in women's health, pregnancy, and childbirth. To avoid wait times for elective services or to receive better accommodations in private facilities,

UNITED KINGDOM'S UNIVERSAL HEALTH CARE SYSTEM

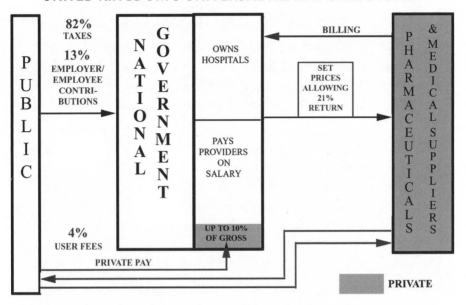

Figure 7.3 - A repeat of the bottom portion of Figure 6.1, the diagram shows the flow of billings (to the left) and payments (to the right) in the United Kingdom health care system. This inexpensive system costs 31 percent of that per capita in the United States. WHO rates it in 18th place overall. Compare with Figures 7.1, p. 122, and 7.2, p. 131.

patients are allowed to pay directly for private care. Owing to the low level of health care funding in the United Kingdom, there is a shortage of both physicians and hospital beds.[124]

The United Kingdom spends the least portion of its Gross Domestic Product on health care of any of the countries considered here, yet its WHO ranking is considerably above that of the United States, which spends more than twice as much. Figure 7.3, duplicated in the previously presented Figure 6.4, shows a diagram of billing and payments in the system. Comparison with the top portion of Figure 6.4, Figure 7.1, and Figure 7.2 shows that the United Kingdom's health care system is the simplest of all. The system does not fix drug prices in the fashion of the other countries, but it limits the profits the pharmaceutical companies make to 21 percent of investment.

Because the United Kingdom's healthcare system is government operated, it is easy to assume that the government not only pays for most health care but decides what health care to provide. However, even though they are employed by the government, it is the country's physicians who, collectively, make most of the decisions regarding what health care to give and who should receive it.[125] Thus the United Kingdom's physicians may actually have more say than their American counterparts who relegate many of the decisions of this sort to insurance issuers, both public and private for-profits.

British physicians tend to devote more resources toward the palliative care of terminal patients than to extreme life-extending surgeries such as kidney transplants and stem cell therapy. When they do resort to such efforts, the costs are far lower than in the United States: $21,000 for kidney transplants in the United Kingdom versus $95,000 to $115,000 in the U.S, and for umbilical cord stem cell transplants $75,000 in the UK versus $334,000 in the U.S.[126]

Germany

Ranked 25th in overall performance, Germany's universal healthcare system derives 90 percent of its funding through social security taxes.[127] The proportion between employer and employee contribution depends on the salary level: the lower the salary, the less the employee contribution. The system also subsidizes health care for the poor and the elderly. The system feeds collected money into nonprofit 'sickness' funds organized according to geographic regions or by trades. These funds compete, but cannot discriminate, and they must all pay for services at the same rates. The richer of the funds are required to contribute to a national pool that doles the money out to the poorer funds. A governing body composed of employers, unions, medical providers, and government personnel sets the rates for hospitals and physician fees. The federal and state governments build the hospitals, but the sickness funds pay for their operation on what amounts to a fee-for-service basis. All physicians belong to associations that receive per capita funding from the sickness funds. These associations pass the money out to the participating physicians on a fee-for-service basis. Germans earning more than a certain amount per year are allowed to opt out of the public system and to carry private insurance that pays providers at a higher rate than allowed by the public system. Very few opt out, however.[128] Recently, the system has instituted co-pays for those of sufficient means. General practitioners operate on a fee-for-service basis, with fees set by a central authority.[129] Most German hospitals (90 percent) are owned by municipalities or religious organizations, and 10 percent are privately owned.[130] One source states that although the German healthcare system is highly fragmented, "The right to health care is regarded as sacrosanct. Universality of coverage, comprehensive benefits, the principle of the healthy paying for the sick, and a redistributive element in the financing of health care have been endorsed by all political parties and are secured in the Basic Law."

Summary

Table 7.2 (in two parts) somewhat summarizes the above discussion and presents additional characteristics of the healthcare systems of these countries and of Canada and the United States.

The table contains these facts regarding the six countries:

- Of the six, the United States has the worst rated healthcare system.
- In terms of percentage of Gross National Product expended, the United States healthcare system is the most expensive by far.
- In terms of expenditure per capita, the United States is the highest by far.
- The United States has a far lower proportion of public to private spending than in the other countries.

Table 7.2 - Numerical characteristics of the six countries considered here. The numbers are from the World Health Organization Report 2000, and represent the situation in 1997.

Country	Overall System Performance Rating	Total Spending as Percent of GNP	Total Spending per Capita (US$)	Percent Spending by Public Sector	Universal Coverage	Percent Population with Public Insurance
France	1st	9.8%	$2,369	76.9%	Yes	99.5%
Japan	10th	7.1%	$2,373	80.2%	Yes	100%
U. K.	18th	5.8%	$1,303	96.9%	Yes	100%
Germany	25th	10.5%	$2,713	77.5%	Yes	92.2%
Canada	30th	8.6%	$1,730	72.0%	Yes	100%
USA	37th	13.7%	$4,187	44.1%	No	45.0%

Table 7.2 Continued - Data for 1997 from World Health Organization and other sources.[131, 132]

Country	Medical Fees Regulated	Expected Life Span (Years)	Infant Mortality per 1000	Hospital Beds per 1000	Physicians/ Nurses per 1000	MRI/ Other Scanners per million
France	Yes	73.1	4.8	8.4	3.3/5.9	9.7/2.5
Japan	Yes	74.5	3.7	16.4	2.0/7.4	69.5/18.8
U. K.	Yes	71.7	5.9	4.1	2.1/4.5	6.3/3.4
Germany	Yes	70.4	4.8	9.2	3.3/9.5	17.1/6.2
Canada	Yes	72.0	6.0	3.9	2.1/7.6	8.1/1.7
USA	No	70.0	7.8	3.6	2.7/8.3	26.9/16.0

- ▶ The United States is the only country without universal healthcare coverage.
- ▶ The United States has far and away the smallest proportion of the population with public healthcare insurance.
- ▶ The United States is the only country that does not regulate fees charged by healthcare providers.
- ▶ The United States has the lowest longevity of the six nations considered.
- ▶ The United States has the highest rate of infant mortality.
- ▶ The United States has the fewest hospital beds per capita.

- France and Germany have more physicians and nurses per capita than the United States but Japan, the United Kingdom and Canada have fewer.
- Japan has far and away the most MRI machines and other scanners. The United States is in second place, and Germany in third. By comparison, France, Canada, and the United Kingdom have very few.

These facts and the other material regarding national healthcare systems that is presented in this chapter show that significant differences exist between countries, both regarding the methodology of providing health care and philosophy— particularly the question of whether health care is a basic right or a privilege.

103. World Health Organization, World Health Report 2000, Health Systems: Improving Performance, Geneva, Switzerland, 215 pp.; www.who.int/whr/2000/en/.

104. Hackney, David, and Debra Rogen, A single payer health care system for the U.S., American Medical Student Association, November 20, 2005.

105. Taylor, Donald H., Jr., What price for-profit hospitals? *Canadian Medical Association Journal*, May 28, 2002; 166 (11); www.cmaj.ca/cgi/content/full/166/11/1418.

106. Steinhauser, Paul, Giulani attacks Democratic health plans as 'socialistic,' CN.com/politics, July 31, 2007; www.cnn.com/2007/POLITICS/07/31/giuliani.democrats/index.html#cnnSTCText.

107. Physicians for a National Health Program (PNHP),International Health Systems; www.pnhp.org/facts/international_health_systems.php?page=4 .

108. LeBow, Robert H., *Health Care Meltdown* (Chambersburg, Pennsylvania, Alan C. Hood & Company, Inc., 2004) p. 144.

109. Ibid, p. 149.

110. Relman, Arnold, Canada's romance with market medicine, Canadian Health Coalition; www.healthcoalition.ca/relman-prospect.html.

111. Woolhandler, S., et al., Costs of heath care administration in the United States and Canada, *The New England Journal of Medicine*, Vol 249, 2003, p. 771.

112. Geyman, John P, *The Corporate Transformation of Health Care* (New York, Springer Publishing Company, 2004), p. 231.

113. Reinhardt, Uwe, et al., Cross-national comparisons of health systems using OECD data, 1959, *Health Affairs*, Vol. 21, No 1, 2002, p. 170.

114. Himmelstein, David U., and Steffie Wollhandler, Why the United States needs a single payer health system, Physicians for a National Health Program, June 29, 1995; www.pnhp.org/facts/why_the_us_needs_a_single_payer_health_system.php.

115. Chua, Kao-Ping, Waiting lists in Canada: Reality or hype?; www.amsa.org/studytours/WaitingTimes_primer.pdf.

116. Statistics Canada, Health Care in Canada, First Annual Report 2000; www.statcan.ca/english/freepub/82-222-XIE/82-222-XIE2000000.pdf.

117. Sanmartin, Claudia, et al., Waiting for medical services in Canada: lots of heat, but little light, *Canadian Medical Association Journal*, Vol. 162, No. 9, May 2, 2000; www.cmaj.ca/cgi/content/full/162/9/1305.

118. Katz, S. J., et al., Phantoms in the snow: Canadians' use of health care in the United States, *Health Affairs*, Vol. 21, No. 1, May-June 2002, pp 19-31.

119. Canadian Institute for Health Information, Understanding emergency department wait times, January 2007; http://secure.cihi.ca/cihiweb/en/downloads/emergency_department_wait_times_e.pdf.

120. Canadian Institute for Health Information, More than half of emergency department visits classified as "Less-urgent" or "Non-urgent;" www.cihi.ca/cihiweb/dispPage.jsp?cw_page=media_14sep2005_e.

121. Klein, Ezra, Health Care Wrapup, April 25, 2005; http://ezraklein.typepad.com/blog/health_of_nations/.

122. World Health Organization, World Health Report 2000, Health Systems: Improving Performance, Geneva, Switzerland, 215 pp.; www.who.int/whr/2000/en/.

123. Ward, Johanna, and Cyntia M. Piccolo, Healthcare in Japan; www.medhunters.com/articles/healthcareInJapan.html.

124. Grant, Sue, Healthcare in the United Kingdom; www.medhunters.com/articles/healthcareInTheUK.html.

125. Aaron, J. Henry, William B. Schwartz, and Mellisa Cox, *Can We Say No?* (Washington, D.C.: Brookings Institution Press, 2005) p. 28.

126. Loc cit, pp. 34 and 54.

127. Hohman, Jessica A., International healthcare systems primer, The American Medical Student Association, 2005; www.amsa.org/uhc/IHSprimer.pdf.

128. Klein, Ezra, *Health Care Wrapup*, April 25, 2005; http://ezraklein.typepad.com/blog/health_of_nations/.

129. National Coalition on Health Care, Health care in Germany; www.nchc.org/facts/Germany.pdf.

130. The Danish Ministry of Health, Hospital, Funding and Casemix, 1999; www.sst.dk/upload/hospital_funding_and_casemix_drg.pdf.

131. NationMaster.com>Health Statistics>Hospital beds (latest by country); www.nationmaster.com/graph-B/hea_hos_bed.

132. NationMaster.com, Health>Statistics>Practicing physicians (latest available) by country; www.nationmaster.com/graph-B/hea_pra_phy.

*To criticize one's country is to do it
a service and pay it a compliment.
It is a service because it may spur
the country to do better than it is
doing; it is a compliment because
it evidences belief that the country
can do better than it is doing.*

—WILLIAM FAULKNER

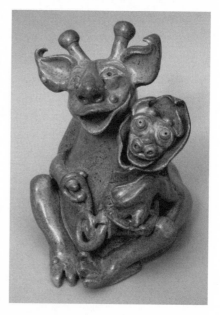

How to Fix the American Health Care System

Every once in a while, I find myself wondering what our incredibly expensive healthcare system really accomplishes for us. I remember that my grandmother, a tough lady who, because there was not enough room for her in the covered wagon along with her seven younger siblings, had walked across a big part of the United States when she was a girl and had never had any medical care until, at age 85, she entered a hospital for the first time and died there. On the other hand, while in his fifties, her father had stuck a pitchfork in his leg, and soon died of blood poisoning because he did not get medical care. It seems that good health and longevity are mostly a matter of genes and luck, plus a modicum of lifestyle. At least that is the way it used to be.

Only during the last half-century has medical care grown to become a significant part of our lives in this country and, simultaneously, transformed itself into a largely corporate enterprise. There can be little doubt that the expansion and increasing availability of health care in the United States has improved our lives and given many of us longer ones. Centenarians are much more common than they used to be. Nevertheless, virtually everyone discussing the American healthcare system now openly admits that the system needs fixing. Views of how to accomplish that end vary considerably.

The View from the Right and Who Promotes It

The view from the right is that the answer to fixing the system is to rely upon what are called "market-oriented solutions" to the healthcare problem. The basic idea is that private enterprise unfettered by government regulation best serves the public interest. Proponents call for minimizing government involvement in health care, and they use in the argument various terms to describe presumably desirable consequences: "greater reliance on personal responsibility," improved "freedom of choice," more "individual liberty" and "accountability," and "a return to traditional American values," involving "democratic capitalism."

Among the more vocal organized opponents of government involvement in health care are various right-wing think tanks, trade associations, and industry front groups. They include the Cato Institute, the Heritage Foundation, the Council for Affordable Health Insurance, the National Center for Policy Analysis, Citizens for Better Medicine, and United Seniors Association.

The Cato Institute is a nonprofit libertarian think tank that "seeks to broaden the parameters of public policy debate to allow consideration of the traditional American principles of limited government, individual liberty, free markets and peace."[133, 134] Cato promotes privatization of government services such as Social Security and Medicare. It receives most of its financial support from individual donations and subscriptions, and has support from large pharmaceutical donors including Eli Lilly & Company, Merck & Company, and Pfizer, Inc.

The Heritage Foundation is perhaps the most influential nonprofit right-wing think tank. The foundation states that its mission is "to formulate and promote conservative public policies based on the principles of free enterprise, limited government, individual freedom, traditional American values, and a strong national defense."[135, 136]

The Council for Affordable Health Insurance is a research and advocacy association of insurance carriers with a membership that includes insurance companies, small businesses, providers, nonprofit associations, actuaries, insurance brokers, and individuals. It is an active advocate for market-oriented solutions to the problems in America's healthcare system.

The National Center for Policy Analysis is a right-wing think tank with programs devoted to promoting privatization in several issue areas, including Social Security, Medicare, and all other health care. The center states that it is a nonprofit, nonpartisan public policy research organization, with its goal to develop and promote private alternatives to government regulation and control, solving problems by relying on the strength of the competitive, entrepreneurial private sector.[137]

Allied with these organizations are others such as The Citizens for Better Medicine, a front group founded by the Pharmaceutical Research and Manufacturers of America (PhRMA). Its function is to protect privatization's interest through advertising, lobbying and congressional contributions.[138] Another front group is the United Seniors Association, which professes to represent older Americans' interests but is primarily a lobbying agent for PhRMA.[139, 140]

On the opposite side of the fence are a number of so-called left-leaning organizations that also profess to be acting in the public interest, but do not go along with the idea that privatization of health care is the answer to the nation's serious health care problem. They include Public Citizen, Center for American Progress, the Brookings Institute, and the Urban Institute, plus a long list of others.

A number of organizations are promoting universal health care; among them is the Physicians for a National Health Program (PNHP), a 14,000-member group of physicians and other healthcare professionals.[141] Joining them in recent months in their arguments for serious healthcare reform that involves greater government involvement are a host of other organizations and persons using the internet to express unhappiness especially with the performance of private for-profit insurers in the health care arena, justifiably so, it seems to me, having read much material presented by both sides. I must admit that my body naturally leans sinistrally, but I find that much of the right-wing pro-private industry argument to be disingenuous in that it is full of what medical author John P. Geyman calls disinformation.[142] The right-wing treatises present some facts, but only those that seemingly bolster their arguments, and those countering are omitted. It's what I call intellectual dishonesty.

Although the pro-privatization forces often claim that their goal is 'affordable health care for everyone,' their real goal is to make health care more affordable to industry and profitable to the insurance element. Not willing to state these goals openly, the pro-privatization forces hide their efforts behind a smokescreen of carefully chosen terminology. Such terms as 'consumer-driven health care,' 'freedom of choice,' 'traditional American values' and 'greater individual responsibility' sound good, but are merely phrases that really mean placing more of the risk burden on the minority group of Americans that consumes most of the health care. The right wing offers no substantive solutions to the health care problem beyond claiming that private enterprise is good for America, government is bad, and therefore private enterprise, not government, should dominate health care. We should just turn health care over to unregulated private enterprise, and that will automatically provide affordable health care for everyone.*

Health care has several major characteristics that make it an unsuitable commodity in the marketplace. A functioning market depends upon the buyers' ability to pick and choose among sellers and the amounts, quality, and quantity they buy—and the sellers' ability to offer products competitively in order to provide the buyers with what they want—in short, a properly functioning marketplace is predicated on the balancing of supply and demand. However, health care needs are characteristically unpredictable and catastrophic, as our family well knows. If we consider the consumers of health care to be the buyers, they have little control over when they need and how much health care they want or need. A family can go into the marketplace to buy food, clothing, or housing and in these arenas make choices based on knowing how much is needed and how much the family can afford. Not so with health care; the family's need is not predictable, nor is the family able to relate its need to family finances because of the often-catastrophic nature of accident and serious illness. The healthcare consumers requiring the most health care simply are not in position to deploy demand market forces that balance the forces associated with supply.

---

* If you believe that, in Alaska we've got a couple of fairly famous bridges you might be interested in buying: our pork-barrel "Bridges to Nowhere," much in the national news in 2007, but not yet built.

Pro-privatization proponents evidently choose to ignore this truth, while simultaneously refusing to face up to the consequences of the medical version of the 80/20 rule: twenty percent of the public will always consume eighty percent of the healthcare burden. Providing that twenty percent the greater choice that consumer-driven health care supposedly engenders and asking it to take on greater personal responsibility makes no sense whatsoever. It's akin to expecting an elephant to fly, an obvious impossibility.

Other Views and Approaches to the Health Care Problem

Happily, we are seeing an increasing level of concern for the problems of the American healthcare system—and a few proposals. Almost daily, newspapers, magazines, and television—and now even the movie *SiCKO*—are devoting attention to the general problem. Politicians running for public office are discussing the issue, and many states are either considering or enacting legislation intended to deal with the problems of high cost and the many Americans without health insurance.

Unfortunately, many of the solutions being proposed are patchwork fixes that fail to address the basic causes of dysfunction in the system. Worse yet, they are even counterproductive to the goal of lowering the overall cost of health care and improving its effectiveness. The fundamental problem is that we have allowed the American healthcare system to become overly dependent upon for-profit private enterprises. Because the primary emphasis of such entities is on creating profit for shareholders, rather than on providing health care, these enterprises are incapable of providing high-quality health care at reasonable cost.

A telling indicator of that fact is provided by the 2007 listing of America's best hospitals published by *U.S. News & World Report* in the July 23/July 30 issue. This listing contains 173 hospitals judged to provide the best care (out of 5,462 examined) in various specialty categories. As nearly as I can determine, not a single one of these 173 is a for-profit hospital. All of them are private nonprofits. Obviously, for-profit hospitals are proving themselves unable to provide the best quality health care, despite their generally higher pricing structures.

Hospitals are a necessary and important part of any health care system, but we have allowed another totally unnecessary component of the system—the for-profit private insurance industry—to take on a dominant role. The industry siphons off a substantial part of the health care dollar while contributing nothing directly to delivery. Furthermore, it too often takes away from medical providers and patients the decision on what medical care to provide.

Years ago, prior to the pervasive development of employer-sponsored insurance purchased from for-profit insurers and operators of health maintenance organizations, the primary decision makers were the physicians and their patients, the actual producers and users of health care. They were the sellers and buyers of health care. Now, the physicians and patients are largely relegated to the background, and the employers have become the buyers and the insurance industry the sellers.[143] Their interests do not coincide with the interests of the providers and users of health care, and that is a fundamental reason why proposed fixes to our health care system based on the private marketplace and for-profit corporations are of no value, and will even make the situation worse. Yet it is easy for politicians and others involved in government to be misguided by the idea that private companies and competition can cut costs and provide adequate health care. They cannot; they only add to the system's fragmentation, high administrative cost, and unsatisfactory health care.[144] Anyone who thinks that marketplace medicine is the answer to America's health care problems should read documentation on the sorry performance of for-profit corporations, "The Health Care Marketplace in the USA," available on line.[145] The site contains a litany of unsavory corporate misdeeds that occur when health care becomes a commodity in the marketplace.

A new book by Harvard economist Katherine Swartz titled *Reinsuring Health*[146] contains what appears to be the inconsistent if not self-contradictory suggestion that the private health industry needs to be retained but that the government should step in and take over the risk involved in paying for the care of those persons who consume the most health care. It is an odd application of the 80/20 rule: basically, the government should insure the insurers for the costly 20 percent of consumers and leave the for-profit insurance industry alone to sell to and profit from the 80 percent who consume the least amount of health care. To put it another way: the government should subsidize the private insurance industry. I am sure the health insurance industry loves this idea—it does nothing to lower overall healthcare costs, but it does guarantee high profit for the insurance industry.

Unfortunately, the concept of reliance on for-profit insurance is so engrained in the public consciousness that most of the proposals for solving the problem of the uninsured are like Swartz's in that they directly incorporate for-profit insurance in the solution. Perhaps even those politicians and others who recognize that for-profit insurance is near the heart of the problem, rather than being a proper part of the solution, are afraid to attack this reality for fear of raising the ire of lobbyists and losing campaign contributions. The consequence is that state and other efforts intended to decrease the number of uninsured—because they typically require citizens to purchase insurance from little-regulated for-profits—have no hope of actually decreasing healthcare costs. Providing "affordable insurance" to everyone is often stated as the well-meaning objective, but it is the wrong objective. Instead, our objective should be to achieve effective, affordable health care to everyone. For us to reach that goal we must heavily regulate for-profit enterprises such as health insurers and pharmaceutical companies and relegate the for-profit insurance industry to a minor role.

All other modern countries have managed to develop more effective and less expensive healthcare systems than we have in the United States. We can do it too.

My Solution

In the search for a viable solution to the American health care problem, I think it is useful to look at those parts of the healthcare system that work the best as well as those that perform poorly and contribute much to the high cost of health care. The formerly much-vilified Veterans Administration healthcare system has so transformed itself during the past two decades that some observers suggest it is a model to be followed. Recently, the president of the Institute for Healthcare Improvement,[†] Donald M. Berwick, said, "If you take a five- or six-year perspective, I think what the Veterans Health Administration has done is stunning. It's especially impressive because this massive system that works in a fishbowl, is under tremendous scrutiny and has constrained resources."[147] The VA has accomplished its transformation by trimming bureaucracy while increasing the number of veterans served, and by integrating services and making heavy use of modern computer technology. While riddled with complexity that needs to be reduced, two other government programs, Medicare and Medicaid, have also served the public well by providing healthcare safety nets for the aged and the poor. These three— Veterans Health Administration, Medicare, and Medicaid—are the best, most cost-effective, parts of the American healthcare system.[‡] The fact that they are all government programs should tell us something about the path we need to follow. With that in mind, and considering the other information portrayed in Table 7.2 and its related descriptions of America's and other national healthcare systems, certain conclusions seem obvious regarding the characteristics of an affordable, effective healthcare system.

---

† The Institute for Healthcare Improvement is a nonprofit organization with broad support from foundations and industry, including insurance companies.

‡ Less cost-effective, and of totally different nature, is the Federal Employees Health Benefits Program (FEHB) through which the federal government pays 75 percent of the cost of private insurance provided by more than 350 commercially available health plans. Eligible for coverage are the president and vice president, members of Congress, federal employees, retirees, former employees, family members, and former spouses—a total of over 9 million people. (U.S. Office of Personnel Management, FEHB Handbook, 2007, www.opm.gov/insure/handbook/fehb01.asp.

ESSENTIAL CHARACTERISTICS

> ▶ *A crucially important characteristic of an effective national health care system is that it must provide comprehensive health care coverage for all its citizens.* If the system does not provide universal coverage, then the poorer elements of society do not get adequate health care. That lack leads to low productivity, low longevity, high infant mortality, and high overall expense in the long run.

> ▶ *The second essential characteristic of an effective health care system is that the cost of providing health care must be distributed to the citizens according to their ability to pay.* To distribute the payment otherwise is to require that the poorest elements of society to pay a higher proportion of their financial resources for health care than the richer elements—and that drives more of a nation's people into poverty.

> ▶ *The third critical element of a good health care system is that the payment for medical services must be uniform*—everyone must be charged equally for what are considered to be necessary health care services, and if there are multiple payers all must pay the same rates.

> ▶ *It is essential that prescription drug prices must be regulated*, either by fixing drug prices or regulating pharmaceutical industry profits.

For a nation to have a health care system with these four essential characteristics, the nation's government must assume the primary role in operating the health care system. Central government control appears to be vital, although the actual operation of the system can be parceled out to regional governments—as in Canada and Germany—or to nonprofit organizations established for the purpose—as in France and Japan. Private, for-profit enterprises can play a role, but this role must be subsidiary to the role of government and not-for-profit private entities. The primary purpose of the health care system must be to provide health care; it cannot be to create profit for the components involved. Certain characteristics of an effective health care system are highly desirable but not absolutely essential:

HIGHLY DESIRABLE CHARACTERISTICS

▸ In the interest of economy, a highly desirable characteristic of a health care system is that it employ a *single payer* for the provision of necessary health care— as in Canada and the United Kingdom. Because a single-payer system allows minimal administrative cost, these two countries have lower per-capita cost than the other countries considered here. If the system is not single-payer, it should at least be all-payer (meaning uniform payment schedules).

▸ The health care system should place *high emphasis on preventive health care*. Failure to do so leads to lower longevity, higher infant mortality, and higher sickness levels that affect the quality of life and the productivity of the work force.

▸ The system's gatekeeper functions should operate in a fashion independent of co-pays. Ideally, *co-pays should be minimized or abolished altogether*, and other mechanisms be instituted to curtail any overuse of the system. The unfortunate thing about co-pays is that they too often discourage timely treatment of health problems.

▸ The system should provide essentially *free or low-cost medical education*. To put the burden on doctors and nurses requires that they seek abnormally high salaries merely to pay off educational debt.

Sadly enough, the United States not only lacks the four essential characteristics of an effective health care system, it has none of what I suggest are four other desirable characteristics. Consequently, the United States has the most expensive and the least effective health care system of any industrialized country. This is a dysfunctional system that is in the throes of total failure—while also growing more expensive by the day. The trend will continue until enough Americans are sufficiently damaged by the system to rise up and demand change.

The truly fundamental problem is the American attitude toward health care. All other modern societies view health care as a human right that their governments have a responsibility to provide, but a substantial portion of the American public is inclined to view health care more as a commodity that can be provided by private enterprise with a minimum of government involvement. Yet, over the past half-century there has been enough recognition of private enterprise's inability to provide an affordable comprehensive health care system that we have created government programs which do provide almost universal health care to certain segments of the population, namely the Medicare, Medicaid, and Veterans Administration segments. These public insurance programs cover approximately 45 percent of the population. The other 55 percent either goes without insurance or depends upon the for-profit private insurance industry.

This is a powerful industry that plays a dominant role in American health care. Its massive lobbying effort, in concert with that of the pharmaceutical industry, has over the years been able to curtail government actions intended to lower health care costs and serve more of the population. The industry's influence extends right down to the personal level by entering into decisions on who gets health care and how much. The term the industry uses to describe payments to providers is a telling indicator of the industry's profit-motivated philosophy; those payouts are called "losses." The private insurance industry absorbs a substantial portion of the American health care dollar because of its high administrative cost and profit-taking. Sadly enough, by looking at the health care systems of other countries, we see that there really is no need for the private health insurance industry even to exist other than perhaps as a minor enterprise serving an elite portion of the public.

What is needed is single-payer universal health care, describable also as universal single-payer public health insurance. The most economical form is a fully socialistic system like the United Kingdom's (and the VA system as well) in which the government owns and operates the hospitals and hires the healthcare providers. Fairly economical also is a capitalistic system akin to Canada's where the provincial governments make global payments to private hospitals and regulated direct fee-for-service payments to providers. Government regulation of pharmaceutical prices or pharmaceutical industry profits also is an essential to reducing the cost of health care.

If we had a king or queen with total power who agreed with the statements in the preceding paragraph, he or she might be inclined to put in place such a system immediately. However, since the current healthcare industry is so large a component of the country's economy (16 percent of Gross National Product), this precipitous action would throw so many people out of work that it probably would create temporary economic chaos.

As desirable as it would be to change the system so drastically in one step, a more pragmatic approach might be to take various individual steps toward the ultimate goal, each step leading directly to that goal:

1—Put in place controls on pharmaceutical prices.

2—Assuming we would retain a fee-for-service system using primarily private healthcare providers, establish set prices (as with Medicare) for all essential medical services and require billing at those prices.

3—Institute a system of global payments to hospitals that requires any for-profit hospitals receive a level of payment equal to that of nonprofit hospitals.

4—Enact laws eliminating tax subsidies to employers for their employee healthcare costs.

5—Extend the age limitations of Medicare downward, perhaps in several steps to cover more of the population, essentially converting it to a universal heath insurance system that would eliminate the need for Medicaid.

6—Enact legislation that would eliminate from the Medicare and Medicaid programs any involvement of for-profit enterprises in administration of those programs.

7—If necessary, increase funding for Medicare sufficiently to allow this program to bear the full costs of the health care of the portion of the populace served.

8—Work toward simplification of the Medicare payment system in ways that will reduce the heavy paperwork load on health care providers.

These actions collectively would substantially lower health care costs by at least 30 percent or more—and bring affordable health care to more—and eventually all—Americans.

It will not be easy, because in there fighting tooth and nail against these changes will be the health insurance and pharmaceutical industries and other organizations dedicated to defending the profitability of their members' operations. Helping them will be the segment of the American population having a high level of mistrust in government and which takes it on faith that private enterprise can best satisfy all of society's needs.

Health care in the United States is not a stand-alone problem. Related is the problem of poverty in this country. The term poverty describes a condition not easily defined and measured, but it alludes to the inability to afford the basic necessities of life. By the most common measure in use—having income less than three times that needed to cover the cost of a nutritionally adequate diet—37 million Americans (13 percent) are living in poverty.[148] In 2006, in the contiguous states, that meant they had incomes less than $9,800 for a single person and less than $20,000 for a family of four. For Alaskans the corresponding amounts were $12,225, and $23,000.[149] With those incomes they can ill afford to pay for more than minimal health care or buy health insurance. A big step forward toward decreasing poverty would be to solve the problem of health care, and the road to solving the health care problem is clearly laid out by the experiences of other countries. It is time for Americans to walk that road while ignoring the blocks laid down by those who assert that the American way is always the best and the propaganda promulgated by vested interests that like things just the way they are while denigrating the best parts of our current system.

We need to remember that no matter how we provide it, health care does not come for free. In the United States individuals pay a high price for health care through a combination of direct payments to providers, purchasing of insurance, and paying taxes. In the other industrialized countries the cost of health care is paid for primarily through taxes, but the rates of taxation vary greatly from country to country. The tax rate for single taxpayers in Japan is much lower than in the United States, the rate in Canada and the United Kingdom is somewhat higher, and the rate in France and Germany is very much higher. In these countries it appears that there is little or no direct connection between taxation rates and the methodology used to pay for their universal health care. And let's remember that these other countries all spend a smaller proportion of their gross national product on health care than does the United States—and do a better job of it.

---

133. Cato Institute, About Us; www.cato.org/about/about.html.

134. People For the American Way, Right Wing Organizations; www.pfaw.org/pfaw/general/default.aspx?oid=4287.

135. People For the American Way, Right Wing Organizations; www.pfaw.org/pfaw/general/default.aspx?oid=4287.

136. The Heritage Foundation, About Us; www.heritage.org/about/.

137. National Center For Policy Analysis; www.ncpa.org/abo/.

138. Public Citizen, United Seniors Association: Hired guns for PhRMA and other corporate interests – July 2002 Report; www.citizen.org/congress/campaign/special_interest/articles.cfm?ID=7999.

139. Public Citizen, United Seniors Association: Hired Guns for PhRMA and Other Corporate Interests - July 2002 Report, www.citizen.org/congress/campaign/special_interest/articles.cfm?ID=7999.

140. Geyman, John P., *The Corporate Transformation of Health Care*, (New York, Springer Publishing Company 2004) p. 181.

141. Physicians for a National Health Program (PNHP); www.pnhp.org/.

142. Geyman, John P., Myths and memes about single-payer health insurance in the United States: a rebuttal to conservative claims, *International Journal of Health Services*, Vol. 35, No. 1, 2005.

143. Richmond, Julius B., and Rashi Fein, *The Health Care Mess* (Cambridge, Massachusetts: Harvard University Press, 2005), p. 137.

144. Moberg, David, More marketplace medicine, *In These Times*, Vol. 24, No 7, 2000; www.inthesetimes.com/issue/24/07/moberg2407.html.

145. The US Marketplace, The health care marketplace in the USA; www.uow.edu.au/arts/sts/bmartin/dissent/documents/health/corporate_overview.html.

146. Swartz, Katherine, *Reinsuring Health* (New York, Russell Sage Foundation, 2007).

147. Gaul, Gilbert M., Revamped Veterans' health care now a model, *Washington Post*, August 22, 2005; www.medicalnewstoday.com/articles/47268.php.

148. Harris, Paul, 37 million poor hidden in the land of plenty, *The Observer*, February 19, 2006; http://observer.guardian.co.uk/world/story/0,,1712965,00.html.

149. 2006 HHS Poverty Guidelines; www.oahhs.org/data/fpl.php.

*We live on through those
lives we have touched.*

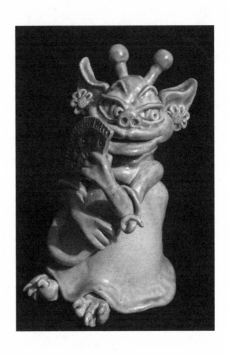

Epilogue: The Rest
of Patricia's Story

This book has described what occurred during the year following Patricia's diagnosis with lung cancer, and what I learned about the American medical system. And so now I tell the rest of the story. I thought I had learned a lot during this trying year for Patricia, but more was to come for both of us.

Each chemotherapy and radiation treatment Patricia received that first year was very tough on her, and for a few days afterward she felt terrible. Nevertheless, she bounced back each time, and throughout retained a cautious optimism. That optimism seemed well justified because by midyear 2005 her x-rays were showing decreasing signs of cancer, and finally none at all. Her hair grew back in, it appeared that she had been cured, and she began working at her job nearly full time.

Having been confined for so long, she was eager to get out more, and as part of that effort we took her in our motor home on a trip to visit a long-time friend in southern Alaska. Not able to do much walking, she wanted to get out into the countryside more and became interested in traveling by four-wheeler on some of the trails around her home in Ester, Alaska. So an arrangement was made for her to have one available.

In late 2005 she was still having breathing problems and they were getting a bit worse. Her oncologist told her that the problem was not the lung cancer but rather an unrelated condition. I wondered about this, and I think Patricia did too. Was the doctor not telling her all he knew simply to help her keep her hopes up? The condition did not improve, and in mid-January 2006 it was clear that she was in trouble. Patricia underwent a needle biopsy and a scan having results that she did not want to discuss, but said the scan had revealed pleural thickening (thickening of the thin serous membrane that covers the lung and lines the chest cavity). That was making breathing difficult for her. In early February her lung was filling with fluid, and a procedure to drain the fluid helped her a great deal, at least enough for her to begin a series of chemotherapy treatments using newly available drugs that her oncologist was able to procure from the manufacturer at no cost to Patricia.

The new drug injections laid her low again, and after a few days there was need to drain more fluid from her lung. She was put in the hospital for several days where a surgeon emplaced a drain in her lung and attempts were made to control the seepage into her lung. That helped her breathing to improve and she returned home. But on February 17 when we visited her she was having enough trouble breathing that we and her live-in companion took her to the hospital emergency room, and she again was admitted to the hospital. There, a surgeon attempted to control the seepage and help healing by several times inserting talcum powder in between the lung and the chest wall. After the last of these procedures, I met the surgeon in the hallway outside her room and he told me that Patricia's lung cavity was badly scarred and that she would be wheelchair-bound and need to be on oxygen continuously "from here on out." I interpreted that to be an ominous statement, but kept the quoted portion of it to myself, as I did not think the surgeon had said that part to Patricia or to anyone else in the family, nor did they need to hear it.

Because Patricia needed to be in a wheelchair meant that she could no longer stay in her house. It was a small older house of substandard construction with small doorways and uneven floors. We lived but a few miles away in a house that we had built with wheelchair access in mind should the need ever arise, and we had a spare bedroom with a convenient adjacent bathroom of moderate size. So when Patricia left the hospital in February she came to stay with us, and she quit her job.

We rented an oxygen separator and she had a portable oxygen bottle to use when going to medical appointments and for emergency use should we have a power failure. Patricia was very concerned about the oxygen supply so, partly for her peace of mind, I set up an emergency generator on our porch where I could immediately connect it to the oxygen separator should we lose power, as we occasionally did for short periods.

Patricia insisted that this was a temporary arrangement and that after some weeks she would be able to return home. Her breathing improved enough that she began going off the oxygen for short periods, and even using a walker on occasion. She was again getting a series of weekly chemotherapy treatments that did not seem to knock her quite so low as before, perhaps in part because her oncologist was also giving her steroids and medications to build up her anemic blood.

As March progressed, Patricia seemed to be doing very well. She spent time working on her various papers, I helped her with her income taxes, and she was spending a few hours on most days working in my wife's pottery studio. She applied her ingenuity and artistic skills toward creating hand-molded gargoyle-like figures, completing more than twenty of them during the next few months. She called them her "Chemo-brain Series," and examples of them and her silversmithing appear throughout this book.

It was obvious that Patricia wanted to be in control of her life as much as possible, and she seemed quite capable of doing so. For that reason I backed off a bit on trying to handle her affairs. Later, I concluded that this was a mistake, that Patricia was not really as capable as she appeared, and that her dealings with health providers and government agencies were especially stressful for her.

Dealing with Medicare and Medicaid

Early on, in late 2004, a nurse at the Fairbanks Memorial Hospital had suggested to Patricia that she might qualify for Medicaid, and so she had applied. After a few months she was informed that she did not qualify because her part-time job (she was working as much as she was physically able) was earning her more than the $200 per month allowed. Furthermore, she had a small IRA funded by money she had inherited, and that was not permissible. The only allowed possessions were a house and a car.

The issue of possible government aid came up again in early 2006. Patricia now had in hand a document signed by her oncologist stating that she was permanently disabled. She was informed that this meant that she might qualify for Medicare, and if that were the case she would qualify for Medicaid as well. Federal Medicare and state Medicaid personnel interviewed her by telephone several times. After each interview she was exhausted and usually in tears, and seeing this I concluded that I should once again get more involved in her financial affairs.

By the time I did again become seriously involved, I discovered that the Medicare and Medicaid people had given Patricia some very bad advice, and that she had followed it. They had apparently assured her that she would qualify for both Medicare and Medicaid, but first she had to get rid of her IRA. They claimed it did not matter by what means she got rid of the money as long as she ended up with no possessions other than her house and car. The result was that Patricia cashed in the IRA to purchase a newer vehicle, using her old car as part of the payment.

But the worst advice she got from the government personnel was regarding her health insurance policy that had become effective in October 2005. However, it did not allow for pre-existing conditions. Medicare and Medicaid would take care of everything, the people told her, so there was no reason to continue the policy when Patricia terminated her job in February 2006, realizing that she could not continue, even on a part-time basis. Interestingly enough, this policy had paid for some of her prescription drugs when Patricia presented the policy information to a pharmacist. She had pointed out that the policy did not allow for pre-existing conditions, but was told not to worry about that because the insurance company would not be able to determine if the prescriptions did or did not relate to a preexisting condition. Patricia followed the bad advice and dropped the policy when she terminated her job. Furthermore, she had never informed the local hospital or her various medical providers that the policy was in effect from October 2005 to March 2006. She just assumed that it would not pay for hospital or provider services. I discovered all this in April 2006.

I first contacted the Social Security office to ask if they did have a completed application from Patricia for Medicare assistance, presenting to the person there proof of power of attorney giving me the right to represent Patricia. No, the power-of-attorney document was not acceptable, I was told, and the office would give me no information other than the fact that if a completed application were in hand the normal processing time would likely be two years. I then found in Patricia's papers verification that a completed application had been received.

People at the local Alaska office handling Medicaid applications were more helpful. Yes, they had an application from Patricia, but they needed more information about her current situation. The power of attorney I had in hand would allow me to represent Patricia, and a representative would interview me. On my several visits to the office I gained the impression that the state people were trying to be helpful, but I also found the whole process was somewhat demeaning. It's no fun to grovel, and I could understand why Patricia cried after (and sometimes during) each Medicare and Medicaid interview. During my main Medicaid interview I explained that Patricia was unable to live at home at least temporarily, and that she was staying at our house. Not long afterwards, I received a letter stating that Medicaid assistance was denied because Patricia was now a member of our household and this household had higher than the allowed $200 per month income.

By this time I had come to understand that the Medicaid program is intended only to serve people who are truly destitute and have no place else to turn. It is not intended to help people like Patricia who could receive help from family or friends.

In fact, just before receiving the denial letter I had decided to withdraw Patricia's application for Medicaid, in part because of the hold the state of Alaska would have on Patricia's estate. By federal law, each state is required to try to recover any Medicaid funds awarded from the estate of the awardee. Patricia owned a house and a car, and if she received any Medicaid funding whatsoever, the state would have first rights to both—to the extent of the aid given. Being a realist, Patricia was well aware that her lifetime might be limited, and she much wanted to make sure that her one granddaughter would have funds available for college. She wrote in her will the provision that her house would serve that end. Wanting to honor that desire, I had decided to withdraw the Medicaid application just as the application was denied.

The sad part of this is that the federal Medicare and state Medicaid people had misled Patricia into thinking that in her situation she would receive aid and therefore should cancel her insurance policy and rid herself of possessions other than house and car. It evidently was going to take up to two years for Medicare to make a decision, and, even if it was positive and made retroactive, that was going to leave Patricia in limbo for a long time. Perhaps, I thought, it does not really take two years to make such a simple decision. Could it be that the two-year wait is in at least part intended to eliminate the need to deal with applicants who do not live that long? No doubt many do not.

Dealing with Hospitals and Insurance Companies

For me, the unpleasant experience with Medicare and Medicaid merely reinforced the earlier lesson that in the affairs of medical finance, the pace of events does not favor the patient. Insurance companies benefit financially by delaying paying out their 'losses.' Likewise, the longer an agency or medical organization can delay on deciding on an application for financial assistance, the better the chance that the need for the decision will disappear, for one reason or another. Perhaps the person dies or perhaps he or his representatives go ahead and pay bills out of pocket.

That could have been the case with Patricia's hospital bills. Early in the game Patricia had applied for financial assistance from the two involved hospitals, Providence Hospital in Anchorage and

Fairbanks Memorial Hospital. Providence Hospital personnel claimed to have lost Patricia's first application, and she sent in a duplicate of the original which somehow also disappeared. Several months after the first application Patricia sent in a new one, and that application was approved. Providence discounted its original $4,279 bill by 73 percent, and we paid the remaining $1,149.

The Fairbanks hospital quickly approved Patricia's application for aid. The hospital discounted its original $56,603 billings by 68 percent, and we promptly paid the remainder, $17,803. Then in October 2005 the hospital informed Patricia that she would need to make a new application for discounting any future bills, and on October 13 she submitted the application. Nothing happened for nine months except that Patricia received another $17,000 in non-discounted billings, which I simply put in the "pending" file.

Finally, in June 2006, I took some action. I had just been invited to appear on the radio show "Talk of Alaska" to participate in a discussion of medical care and finances in Alaska. By this time the efforts I had been taking on Patricia's behalf had received some attention locally and even, to a minor extent, nationally. An editor on the nationally distributed monthly *Orthopedics Today* had interviewed me about my experiences in dealing with Patricia's medical bills, and the interview had appeared in the April 2007 issue. So prior to the radio show I wrote a letter to the head of the Fairbanks Memorial Hospital, Mike Powers, telling him that I had been invited to appear on the show to discuss my experiences and that I wished to talk with him before the show to gain any input that he might have. Thinking it might also help to get his attention, I sent him a copy of the *Orthopedics Today* interview. I mentioned in the letter that I would like also to discuss Patricia's unanswered request for financial aid.

Mike Powers granted the interview and was helpful in every way. He answered all of the various questions I put to him on issues that I might discuss in the radio show, and when I turned to the matter of Patricia's application for aid he called in his primary fiscal officer. I had a copy of Patricia's nine-month-old application with me plus all supporting documents, even including her last year's income tax return, which I handed over to the officer.

The result was immediate action on the application and the unexpected cancellation of all of Patricia's medical bills from the hospital from October 2005 onward. Under the circumstances, I thought that the hospital officials were being very generous—they knew that I was prepared to pay any reasonably discounted bills.

But that was far from the end of the story. By this time I had become aware of the health insurance policy that Patricia thought would not cover her hospital or health provider costs because of the pre-existing condition clause.

In a conversation with one of the hospital's fiscal people I mentioned the policy and the person asked me to contact the insurance company about it. I called a representative and described the situation, saying that we were assuming that, because of the pre-existing condition clause, the policy would not cover Patricia's hospital and medical provider expenses. The representative said that was correct, and we terminated the conversation. Then about three hours later she called me back and said, "I have been thinking about our earlier discussion, and of course there is a lot of money involved, but I wonder if some of the coding designations for certain of the recent services Patricia has received might be sufficiently different from those of earlier services that they would be covered. Why don't you suggest that the hospital submit the bills, and we will see."

The result was that the hospital did submit the bills and did receive payment for at least a major portion of what it had agreed to write off. I then contacted Patricia's oncologist and another surgeon who had written off his services with the suggestion that their billings be submitted to the insurance company. The insurance company provided some payment on those billings as well. I am not sure what happened here. Possibly some of the coding had changed, or perhaps the insurance company representative I contacted intervened in a way that caused the company to view the billings as not relating to a pre-existing condition.

I too had made the mistake of assuming that Patricia's policy would not pay for various services she was getting, with the consequence that I spent money unnecessarily. Because the monthly rental was so high, $200 per month, I had replaced the wheelchair the hospital provided with a purchased one. We put out money for refilling oxygen bottles that would have been paid for under the policy, and I had even contemplated buying an oxygen separator because the rent on the one the hospital had provided was so high, $300 per month. In retrospect, it amazes me that I, a person who was paying a great deal of attention to the financial aspects of Patricia's illness, did not recognize all the various fiscal avenues available, nor realize that I should delay in making certain payments to medical providers.

In the meantime, Patricia seemed to be doing quite well. Her spirits were good and she was continuing several days each week to work on her "Chemo-brain Series" of clay figurines. She had been going down a flight of stairs to work in Rosemarie's pottery studio, but when that was difficult we moved a table into the living room for her to work on.

By mid-July Patricia was truly aware that her illness was terminal, and at that time we received visitations from the hospital's Home Care personnel and from the local hospice, the oncologist having contacted them both. Patricia was growing weaker and requiring more medication, including occasional morphine injections.

On the morning of July 31, 2006, I was holding Patricia in my arms as Rosemarie and I were giving her a morphine injection. I felt her whole body suddenly relax, and I knew then that our daughter was dead.

We cannot know for sure, but things might have gone differently if, back in 2004, Patricia had been in a situation where she felt financially able to visit a doctor prior to being in Stage III of her lung cancer at the time of diagnosis.

✤

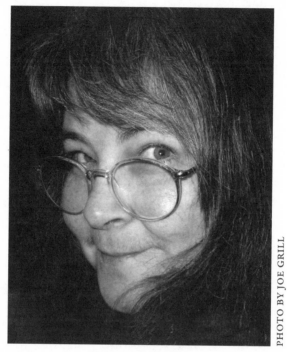

Patricia Ann Davis
1953—2006

In Memoriam
To a Teacher and Artist Who Created
Unique Beauty in All She Touched

Acknowledgements

Two nationally known physicians, orthopedic surgeon Dr. Alan H. Morris of St. Louis, Missouri, a member of the editorial board of *Orthopedics Today*, and Dr. John P. Geyman, former chairman of the Family Medicine Department at the University of Washington School of Medicine, have been particularly helpful to me by reading and discussing parts of the material in this work. Taking much interest also has been Fairbanks obstetrician Dr. Richard Anderson who helped me clarify some of the discussion, and Fairbanks orthopedic surgeon Dr. Richard Cobden who helped point me in the right directions. Fairbanks ophthalmologist Dr. Ronald W. Zamber helped me in the early investigation of CPT coding, and Ruth Benson, RN, read and criticized the manuscript several times along the way. I thank Fairbanks Memorial Hospital CEO Mike Powers of Banner Health and Daniel E. Winfree, executive director of The Greater Fairbanks Community Hospital Foundation, Inc., for providing me with extensive data on the operation of the Fairbanks Memorial Hospital. In the interest of avoiding causing them any possible awkwardness, I refrain from naming the many medical professionals who treated Patricia. They know who they are, and our family thanks them for their compassionate care of our daughter. During the production of this book it has been a pleasure to work with the primary editor, Carla Helfferich of McRoy & Blackburn Publishers, and designer Deirdre Helfferich, managing editor of the Ester Republic Press. They are major contributors. Patricia's sister, Deborah Jo Gonzalez, has contributed many insightful suggestions and helped with proofreading. Rosemarie, my wife for 56 interesting years, has of course been involved from beginning to end. She shares with me the great sense of loss that comes from losing our first-born daughter in this manner, and she has contributed much to the form of this book through discussion and repeated critical readings of the manuscript.

Glossary

Note: A few common terms not referred to in text are contained in this glossary for the benefit of those reading similar works.

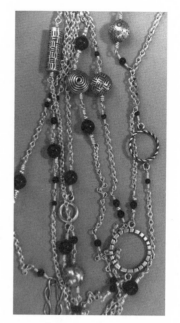

Acronyms

CMI Case Mix (or Case Mix Index)

CMS Centers for Medicare and Medicaid Services

CPT Current Procedural Terminology coding system

DRG Diagnosis Related Group

DSH Disproportionate Share Hospital

EPO Exclusive Provider Organization

FDA Food and Drug Administration

GPCI Geographic Practice Cost Indices

HCFA Health Care Financing Administration

HCPCS HCFA Common Procedural Coding System

HMO Health Maintenance Organization

ICD-9-CM International Classification of Diseases, 9th Edition, Clinical Modification

IME Indirect Medical Education payment

IPA Independent Practice Association

MRI Magnetic Resonance Imaging

NIH National Institutes of Health

PFFS Private Fee-For-Service (Plan)

PhRMA Pharmaceutical Research and Manufacturers of America

PPO Preferred Provider Organization

POS Point-Of-Service (Plan)

PPS Prospective Payment System

RVS (RBRVS) Relative Value Scale or Resource-Based Relative Value Scale

RVU Relative Value Units used in the RBRVS system

SCH Sole Community Hospital

SSI Supplemental Security Income
VA Veterans Administration
UNFC Uniform National Conversion Factor

Actual Bill (Charge) or **Actual Billing** The amount a physician or
other provider actually bills a patient for a particular medical
service, procedure or supply in a specific instance. The actual
charge may differ from (and is typically 2- 4 times larger
than) the usual, customary, prevailing, and/or reasonable
amount the provider expects to be paid by Medicare or
medical insurers. *See also:* **Super Bill** and **Charge Ticket**.

Acute Care Hospital care given to patients who generally require
a stay of up to seven days and that focuses on a physical or
mental condition requiring immediate intervention and
constant medical attention, equipment and personnel.

All-Payer System A system that imposes uniform prices on medical
services, regardless of who's paying. Most or all modern
countries except the United States have either single-payer or
all-payer systems.

Average Wholesale Price (AWP) The price arbitrarily set by
pharmaceutical wholesalers to open negotiations. It almost
always exceeds the average price actually paid.

Base Payment Rate (Standard DRG Payment) The payment per
unit DRG (defined below) to hospitals for Medicare services.
In 2005, it was $4,570.

Capitalism The economic system in which all or most of the means
of production and distribution, as land, factories, railroads,
etc., are privately owned and operated for profit, originally
under fully competitive conditions: it has been generally
characterized by a tendency toward concentration of wealth,
and, in its later phase, by the growth of great corporations,
increased governmental control, etc. (first meaning from
Webster's dictionary). *See also:* **Socialism** and **Nonprofit**.

Capitation The payment for services on a per-head basis, as
contrasted to a fee-for-service basis.

Case Mix Index, or **Case Mix (CMI)** A measure of relative severity of medical conditions of a hospital's patients. It represents the average DRG of all that hospital's patient discharges. If the case mix index is less than 1.0 it means that this hospital's patients, on average, require fewer hospital resources than average, or if the CMI is greater than 1.0 it means that the patients require move than average hospital resources.

Centers for Medicare and Medicaid Services (CMS) An agency of the U.S. Department of Health & Human Services that operates or oversees the Medicare, Medicaid and the State Children's Health Insurance Program. Formerly, it was called the Health Care Financing Administration (HCFA).

Chargemaster A master listing of charges established by a hospital or hospital system that can involve determined charges for as many as 45,000 chargeable items using the ICD-9-CM coding system.

Charge Ticket (or **Super Bill**) An internally developed document that physicians or other medical providers generate to capture the information required to bill Medicare or other insurers for services rendered to patients. *See also:* **Actual Bill**.

Cherry Picking The practice used especially by for-profit insurers of seeking only healthy customers in order to maximize profits.

Coding A mechanism for identifying and defining physicians' and hospitals' services. Coding provides universal definition and recognition of diagnoses, procedures and level of care. Coders usually work in medical records departments and coding is a function of billing. Medicare fraud investigators look closely at the medical record documentation that supports codes and look for consistency. Lack of consistency of documentation can earmark a record as "upcoded" which is considered fraud.

Consumer In the context here, a consumer is a person using healthcare services.

Consumer-Driven Health Care Health care paid for directly and chosen by consumers without the intervention of insurance companies. Although not intended to, the term rightfully includes health care paid for by uninsured persons.

Contract Research Organizations For-profit companies who contract to establish networks of physicians who are paid to administer drugs and collect information during clinical trials. Approximately 1000 are in operation worldwide.

Co-Payment A type of cost-sharing that requires the insured or subscriber to pay a specified flat dollar amount or proportion, usually on a per-unit-of-service basis, with the third-party payer reimbursing some portion of the remaining charges.

Cost Shifting When rates are set higher than actual costs to recover unreimbursed costs from government, uninsured, underinsured and other payers.

Cost-To-Charge Ratio A number derived by dividing the costs a hospital incurred during a pervious accounting period by the chargemaster rates in effect at the time.

Current Procedural Terminology (CPT) A coding system used to determine Medicare reimbursement rates.

Customary, Prevailing, or Reasonable A fee or payment considered to be fair in the context of the community, is reasonable, and falls within the customary range of fees or payments prevailing in a specific geographic area for the provision of a similar service, procedure, or supply. It is often far lower than the actual billing amounts.

Deductible Required out-of-pocket expenditure by the covered individual before the insurer pays towards the allowable charges for a covered service. Deductibles may be specified in dollar amounts or units of service.

Defined Contribution Coverage A funding mechanism for health benefits whereby employers make a specific dollar contribution toward the cost of insurance coverage for employees, but make no promises about specific benefits to be covered.

Diagnosis Related Group (DRG) A hospital classification system that groups patients by common characteristics requiring treatment. More than 500 categories are in use.

Disproportionate Share Hospital (DSH) A hospital that provides care to a high number of patients who cannot afford to pay and/or do not have insurance. Fairbanks Memorial is an example.

Disproportionate Share Payment The payment awarded by Medicare to a hospital that serves more than usual low-income patients.

Downcoding and Bundling The practice by insurers of lowering the codes or grouping together codes for the purpose of minimizing payment to providers.

DRG Weight A multiplier assigned by CMS to each DRG grouping that relates the cost of the DRG to the average cost of all 500+ DRGs across the nation during the previous year or accounting period.

Eighty-twenty (80/20) Rule (also **20/80**, also the **Pareto Principle**, the **Law of the Vital Few**, and the **Principle of Factor Sparsity**) A numerically inexact rule of thumb expressing the idea that most of the effects (80 percent) will come from 20 percent of the causes. It is used in various contexts and applications with sometimes different numerical values, e.g., 90/10. The medical version states that 20 percent of the population will account for 80 percent of healthcare expenses.

Exclusive Provider Organizations (EPOs) Insurance vehicles similar to HMOs but which cover expenses only for services from in-network providers.

Explanation of Medicare Benefits (EOMB) The statement of payment from Medicare; it shows the amount charged by the provider, the amount approved by Medicare and the amount actually paid by Medicare. It is the statement that is submitted to the insurance company for payment under the Medigap policy. Other insurers sometimes use the term explanation of benefits (EOB) to refer to their own payment statements.

Extended Care Facility A nursing home-type setting that offers skilled, intermediate, or custodial care.

False Claims Act A federal law that imposes liability for treble damages and fines of $5,000 to $10,000 for knowingly submitting a false or fraudulent claim for payment to the federal government.

Favorable Selection Strategy used by insurance companies that encourages the enrollment of healthier people while discouraging the enrollment of sicker people. *See also:* **Cherry-picking.**

Federal HMO Act Federal law regulating HMOs. Under the Federal HMO act, an entity must have three characteristics to call itself an HMO: (1) an organized system for providing health care or otherwise assuring health care delivery in a geographic area, (2) an agreed-upon set of basic and supplemental health maintenance and treatment services, and (3) a voluntarily enrolled group of people.

Fee Schedule A comprehensive listing of fees used by either a healthcare plan or the government to reimburse providers on a fee-for-services basis.

Fee-For-Service A method in which physicians and other healthcare providers receive a fee for services performed, receiving payment for specific services provided.

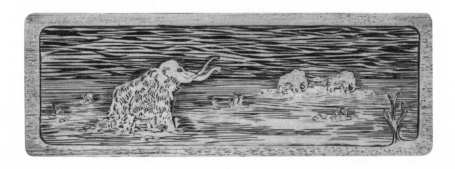

Fee Schedule Payment Area A geographic area within which payments for a given service under the Medicare Fee Schedule will be equal. There are 100 of these in United States; all of Alaska is one.

Fiscal Intermediary (or **Intermediary**) A for-profit insurance company that acts as a regional administrator of payments and reimbursements to hospitals for government programs such as Medicare.

Food and Drug Administration (FDA) The agency within the U.S. Department of health and Human Service responsible for regulating food, dietary supplements, drugs, biological medical products, blood products, medical devices, radiation-emitting devices, veterinary products and cosmetics in the United States.

For-Profit An organization designed to make a profit; one with shareholders: contrasting with nonprofit.

Fortune 500 A listing of the 500 largest corporations in America produced annually by *Fortune* magazine.

Free-Standing Facility Usually a specialty facility that is not part of a comprehensive care system, for example, a free-standing surgery facility or a free-standing assisted living facility.

Free-Standing Outpatient Surgical Center A healthcare facility that is physically separate from a hospital, and that provides pre-scheduled, outpatient surgical services. Also called surgicenter or ambulatory surgical facility.

Freedom of Choice (FOC) In general, laws that permit enrollees to choose any provider and receive substantial reimbursement from their health plan. Also refers to a federal Medicaid rule requiring states to ensure that Medicaid beneficiaries are free to obtain services from any qualified provider. Exceptions are possible through waivers of Medicaid and special contract options.

Gag Clause or **Gag Rule** A provision in a provider contract with a managed care organization or insurer that prevents providers from discussing all available treatment options or financial incentives provided by the insurer with patients.

Gatekeeper A primary care physician responsible for overseeing and coordinating all aspects of a patient's medical care and pre-authorizing specialty care.

General Practitioner Physician whose practice is based on a broad understanding of all illnesses and who does not restrict his/her practice to any particular field of medicine.

Generic (Drug or Substitution) In cases in which the patent on a specific pharmaceutical product expires and drug manufacturers produce generic versions of the original branded product, the generic version of the drug (which is theorized to be exactly the same product manufactured by a different firm) is dispensed even though the original product is prescribed. Some managed care organizations and Medicaid programs mandate generic substitution because of the generally lower cost of generic products.

Geographic Practice Cost Indices, or Geographic Factors (GPCI) Annually adjusted multipliers applied to Relative Value Units to adjust for cost differentials in the 100 designated areas of the United States called Fee Schedule Payment Areas. Specific multipliers pertain to each of the areas, and they apply separately to physician labor, practice, and malpractice insurance costs.

Global, Global Payment Annual payment such as is used in Canada to reimburse hospitals, where it is negotiated between the hospitals and the provincial governments. It is far less cumbersome than fee-for-service payments.

Group Health Insurance Health insurance purchased through a group that exists for some purpose other than buying insurance, such as a workplace, labor union, or professional association.

Group Insurance Any insurance policy or health services contract by which groups of employees (and often their dependents) are covered under a single policy or contract, issued by their employer or other group entity.

Group Practice Association A formal arrangement of three or more physicians or other health professionals providing health services. Income is pooled and redistributed to the members of the group according to a prearranged plan.

Health Care Common Procedural Coding System (HCPCS) Federal coding system for medical procedures. HCPCS includes Level I CPT (Current Procedural Terminology) codes, and Level II codes which supplement the CPT codes. The Level II codes include physical services not included in CPT as well as non-physician services such as ambulance, physical therapy and durable medical equipment. They may be either national or local. The local codes are developed by local Medicare carriers to supplement the national codes. HCPCS codes are five-digit codes, the first digit a letter followed by four numbers. HCPCS codes beginning with A through V are national; those beginning with W through Z are local.

Health Care Financing Administration (HCFA) The federal agency that formerly administered the Medicare, Medicaid and children's health insurance programs prior to its conversion to the Centers for Medicare & Medicaid Services (CMS).

Healthcare Provider An individual or institution that provides medical services.

Health Insurance A mechanism to spread the risk of unforeseen expenditures across a broad base to protect the individual from crippling personal expenditures for healthcare services. Health insurance may be purchased individually or on a group basis. It may be custom designed to cover specific services and procedures and include requirements to control the level of use and payment for these services. An employee health insurance benefit is a nontaxable form of compensation to the employee in lieu of taxable salary or wages, provided through employment. Various types of insurance, such as accident, disability income, medical expense, dental, vision, hearing, and accidental death and dismemberment may be made available through employment. Benefits may be available to dependents of active employees, retirees, spouses, survivors, and dependents through employment. Benefits for classes of active and retired employees and their dependents need not be uniform. The employer may purchase benefits or the costs may be shared between the employer and employee.

Health Maintenance Organizations (HMOs) Entities that offer prepaid, comprehensive health coverage for both hospital and physician services with specific healthcare providers using a fixed structure or capitated rates.

Health Savings Accounts (HSAs) Put in place by a provision of the Medicare Prescription Drug Improvement and Modernization Act of 2003, health savings accounts use individual's pre-tax dollars to pay portions of medical bills, provided that the individual also buys a high-deductible health plan from an insurance company.

High-Deductible Health Plan (HDHP) A type of insurance policy typically cheaper than traditional health insurance by 30 to 50 percent. The HDHP annual deductible must be at least $1,000 for an individual and $2,000 for a family. The annual out-of-pocket expense (including co-pays and deductibles) must not exceed (in 2006) $5,250 for an individual and $10,500 for a family.

Hill-Burton Act Federal legislation enacted in 1946 to support the construction and modernization of healthcare institutions.

Hill-Burton Program Federal program created in 1946 to provide funding for the construction and modernization of healthcare facilities. Hospitals which receive Hill-Burton funds must provide specific levels of charity care.

Home Care In contrast with inpatient and ambulatory care, home care is medical care ordinarily administered in the home setting when a patient is not sufficiently ambulatory to make frequent office or hospital visits. With these patients, intravenous therapy (for example) is administered at the patient's residence, usually by a healthcare professional. Home care reduces the need for hospitalization and its associated costs.

Hospice A facility or program that is licensed, certified or otherwise authorized by law, that provides supportive care of the terminally ill.

Hospice Care Care that addresses the physical, spiritual, emotional, psychological, financial, and legal needs of the dying patient and the family; provided by an interdisciplinary team of professionals and perhaps volunteers in a variety of settings, including hospitals, freestanding facilities, and at home.

Hospital An institution whose primary function is to provide inpatient diagnostic and therapeutic services for a variety of medical conditions, both surgical and nonsurgical. In addition, most hospitals provide some outpatient services, particularly emergency care. Hospitals may be classified by length of stay (short term or long term), as teaching or nonteaching, by major types of services (psychiatric, tuberculosis, general, and other specialties, such as maternity, pediatric, or ear, nose and throat), and by type of ownership or control (federal, state, or local government; for-profit and not-for-profit).

Indirect Medical Education (IME) payment An add-on to the base DRG payment made by Medicare for the purpose of helping to support medical education. It goes only to those hospitals having a teaching function.

Inlier A hospital patient whose length of stay or service cost resembles those of most other patients. See also: outlier.

Inpatient A patient who has been admitted at least overnight to a hospital or other health facility and occupies a hospital bed, crib, or bassinet while under observation, care, and diagnosis. *See also:* **Outpatient**.

Inpatient Services Items and services furnished to a patient staying overnight in a hospital including bed and board, nursing and related services, diagnostic and therapeutic services, and medical or surgical services.

Intermediary (or **Fiscal intermediary**) A for-profit insurance company that acts as a regional administrator of payments and reimbursements to hospitals for government programs such as Medicare.

International Classification of Diseases, 9th Edition, Clinical Modification (ICD-9-CM) The World Health Organization's Ninth Revision, International Classification of Diseases (ICD-9) is the official system of assigning codes to diagnoses and procedures associated with hospital utilization in the United States.

Long-Term Care Care given to patients with chronic illnesses and whose length of stay in a care facility is longer than 30 days.

Long-Term Care Insurance A continuum of maintenance and health services provided to the chronically or mentally ill or the disabled on an ongoing basis.

Magnetic Resonance Imaging (MRI) A diagnostic technique that uses radio and magnetic waves, rather than radiation, to create images of body tissue and to monitor body chemistry.

Major Diagnostic Category (MDC) A clinically coherent grouping of ICD-9-CM diagnoses by major organ system or etiology that is used as the first step in assignment of most diagnosis-related groups (DRGs). MDCs are commonly used for aggregated DRG reporting.

Malpractice A dereliction from professional duty or a failure to exercise an accepted degree of professional skill or learning by one (as a physician) rendering professional services which results in injury, loss, or damage. Also an injurious, negligent, or improper practice.

Managed Care Program A program, typically operated by a for-profit insurance company, that controls all aspects of the health care it provides to its beneficiaries. The programs are of several types: Health maintenance organizations (HMOs), preferred provider organizations (PPOs), and point of service (POS) plans. They receive set payments from Medicare under

Medicare C for their Medicare beneficiaries and accept the financial risk for their care.

Market Area The geographic area over which a product or service is sold and perhaps targeted by insurance companies or other enterprises for greatest market and profit potential.

Market-Based Reform Basically, the privatization of health care for the purpose of maximizing profit—often touted by right-wing components of American society.

Marketplace Medicine The practice of competition for patients among providers and professionals as a profit-making mechanism.

Maximum Allowable Charge The largest dollar amount to which an insurance carrier will apply plan benefits.

Medicaid A federally-funded, state-run program that provides medical assistance for individuals and families with limited incomes and resources. It pays for healthcare costs, including doctor's visits and eye care.

Medical Education and Communication Companies (MECCs) For-profit enterprises hired by pharmaceutical companies to promote their products under the guise of providing education to doctors.

Medical Loss Ratio The portion of money paid into an insurance pool that actually goes to paying for medical benefits. If the ratio is 60 percent, it means 60 percent of the income goes to pay benefits.

Medicare (Title XVIII) Federal program that provides basic health care and limited long term care for retirees and certain disabled individuals without regard to income level. Beneficiaries must pay premiums, deductibles and coinsurance.

Part A - Medicare: hospital insurance that helps pay for medically necessary inpatient hospital care, and, after a hospital stay, limited inpatient care in a skilled nursing facility, for limited home health care or hospice care.

Part B - Medicare: medical insurance that helps pay for medically necessary physician services, outpatient hospital services and supplies that are not covered by the hospital insurance.

Part C - *See* **Medicare Advantage** and **Medicare + Choice**; *also*: **Medicare D**.

Medicare Advantage (formerly called **Medicare + Choice**) Any of several plans operating under Medicare Part C, such as HMOs, PPOs and PFFSs serving patients who have opted out of Medicare A and B.

Medicare Allowance (Medicare Approved Amounts) The total amount that a Medicare Participating Provider can receive for a given CPT Code procedure from a Medicare patient. Medicare normally pays 80 percent of this amount, the other 20 percent coming from the patient or a secondary insurer.

Medicare Carrier A for-profit insurance company that acts as a regional administrator of payments and reimbursements to medical providers submitting billings to Medicare B.

Medicare + Choice (Also referred to as **Medicare Part C** and **Medicare Advantage**) A Medicare program under which eligible Medicare enrollees can elect to receive benefits through a managed care program that places providers at risk for those benefits.

Medicare D A part of the Medicare program that pays part of the cost that Medicare patients pay for prescription drugs. Put in place by the Medicare Prescription Drug Improvement, and Modernization Act of 2003, Public Law 108-173.

Medicare Intermediary (or **fiscal intermediary**) A for-profit insurance company that contracts with the CMS to process payment submissions from hospitals to Medicare A.

Medicare Localities The United States is divided into 100 Medicare localities wherein Medicare payments for provider services are uniform.

Medicare Participating Provider A healthcare provider who agrees to accept Medicare Approved Amounts (Medicare Allowances) from patients covered by Medicare. *See also:* **Nonparticipating Provider** and **Private-pay Contractor**.

Medigap Policy An insurance policy providing supplemental coverage for Medicare patients.

"Me-too" Drugs Drugs that are merely minor variants of existing drugs containing no new active ingredients and which may be no more or even less effective than those already on the market. The only requirement is that they be better than placebos.

National Health Insurance Any federal program that uses tax funds to finance the provision of comprehensive health benefits for the population.

National Institutes of Health (NIH) An agency of the U.S. Department of Health and Human Services. It is the primary federal agency for conducting and supporting medical research.

Nonparticipating Provider A healthcare provider who chooses not to accept Medicare allowances from patients covered by Medicare. Medicare pays nonparticipating providers 95 percent of what it pays participating providers, but they are allowed to collect up to 115 percent of the Medicare Allowance from patients covered by Medicare. *See also:* **Private-pay Contractor**.

Nonprofit, or Not-for-profit Nonprofits do not operate to generate excess income, a characteristic widely considered to be the defining characteristic of such organizations. However, a nonprofit organization may legally and ethically trade at a profit. The extent to which it can generate income may be constrained, or the use of those profits may be restricted. *See also:* **Capitalism**.

Out-of-Pocket Maximum A dollar amount set by an insurance policy that limits the annual total amount (aside from premiums) that the policy holder must expend for medical care that the policy covers.

Outlier A comparative term describing a patient whose stay in the hospital is unusually long or whose costs for hospital care are unusually high compared to other patients with the same diagnosis or condition. The Medicare Part A program uses DRGs as categories to identify outliers. Under Medicare, additional payments are made for outliers meeting certain conditions.

Outpatient A person who receives healthcare services without being admitted to a hospital.

Outpatient Services Medical and other services provided by a qualified facility where an overnight stay is not required, such as therapy and other clinics, labs and diagnostic centers.

Over-the-Counter Drugs Drugs that do not require prescriptions.

Overvalued Procedure A procedure for which the payment rate has been reduced because it was identified as "overvalued" under the customary, prevailing, and reasonable payment system.

Participating Provider A healthcare provider who participates in Medicare or who has a contractual arrangement with a healthcare service contractor, HMO, PPO, IPA or other Managed Care Organization.

Patient Person who is receiving medical care. There are two types of patients: inpatients, who are admitted to hospitals, and outpatients, who are not.

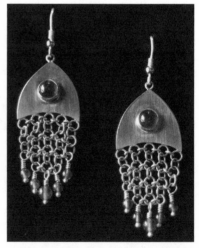

Payer Generally regarded as the guarantor of payment; could be a government entity, an employer, health and welfare fund, insurer, a broker for the employer or labor organization acting in a purchasing agent capacity, or an individual.

Peer Review Organization An organization established to set standards for medically necessary procedures. It is composed of practicing doctors and other professionals.

Pharmaceutical Research and Manufacturers of America (PhRMA) A trade organization representing the pharmaceutical industry. It states its mission is "to conduct effective advocacy for public policies that encourage discovery of new medicines for patients by pharmaceutical/ biotechnology research companies.

Physician's Current Procedural Terminology (PCPT or CPT) A list of medical services and procedures performed by physicians and other providers. Each service and/or procedure is identified by its own unique five-digit code. CPT has become the healthcare industry's standard for reporting physician procedures and services, thereby providing an effective method of nationwide communication. *See also:* **Health Care Common Procedural Coding System (HCPCS).**

Point-of-Service Plans (POSs) Insurance plans similar to HMOs but, like PPOs, allow for payment of services from providers outside the network when the policy holder pays a higher proportion of the provider charges.

Practice Expense The cost of nonphysician resources incurred by the physician to provide services. Examples include salaries and benefits for employees, and the expenses associated with the purchase and use of medical equipment and supplies.

Pre-Existing Conditions When a physical or mental condition of a newly insured individual is present prior to the issuance of the new insurance policy. Normally, these exclusions last from six to twelve months, however, more severe conditions may be considered as lifetime exclusions.

Preferred Provider Organization (PPO) Contractual arrangements among hospitals, physicians, employers, insurance companies, or third-party administrators to provide healthcare services to subscribers at a negotiated, often discounted, price.

Preferred Providers Physicians, hospitals, and other healthcare providers who contract to provide health services to persons covered by a particular health plan.

Preventive Care Comprehensive care emphasizing priorities for prevention, early detection and early treatment of medical conditions, generally including routine physical examination and immunizations.

Primary Care Entry-level care which may include diagnostic, therapeutic or preventive services.

Private Fee-For-Service (Plan) PFFS An insurance plan offered by commercial insurers to persons enrolled in both Part A and Part B of Medicare. Members are allowed to choose any provider that accepts Medicare patients and also agrees to abide by the plan's payment provisions. Such a plan may provide coverage for prescription drugs and certain services beyond those covered by Medicare Parts A and B. The insurer pays providers directly without the intervention of Medicare intermediaries or Medicare carriers.

Private-pay Contractor A healthcare provider who chooses to opt out of Medicare altogether. The provider is not allowed to bill Medicare for any services to any patient, and he can charge the patient anything he chooses.

Proprietary Hospital An investor-owned hospital operated for the purpose of making a profit for its owners. An example is the Alaska Regional Hospital in Anchorage.

Prospective Payment System (PPS) A fee-for-service system established by CMS to pay hospitals for Medicare inpatient care.

Provider Generically, a professional engaged in the delivery of health services, including physicians, dentists, nurses, podiatrists, optometrists, clinical psychologists, etc. Hospitals and long-term care facilities are also providers. The Medicare program uses the term "provider" more narrowly, to mean participating institutions: hospitals, skilled nursing facilities, home health agencies, etc.

Provider-Sponsored Organization (PSO) A provider-owned entity that is certified by HCFA to participate in the Medicare + Choice program and to assume risk for benefits provided to Medicare beneficiaries. Also referred to as Provider Services Organizations.

Qualified Medicare Beneficiary (QMB) A person whose income falls below 100 percent of Federal poverty guidelines and whose resources do not exceed twice the resource limit of the SSI program, for whom the state must pay the Medicare Part B premiums, deductibles and co-payments.

Research and Development In the context here, the activities involved in discovering, testing, and manufacturing drugs in order to bring them to market.

Reasonable and Customary Fee A reasonable fee is a fee that, in the context of the community, is fair. A customary fee is a fee that falls within the customary range of fees prevailing in a specific geographic area for the provision of a similar service, procedure, or supply. It is often far lower than the actual billing to uninsured persons. *See also:* **Customary, Prevailing, or Reasonable**

Redlining An insurance practice used to exclude entire occupations, businesses, geographic areas, and age groups from health insurance coverage for the purpose of limiting loss.

Relative Value Units (RVUs) Units of measure used in the Resource-Based Relative Value Scale. They are applied to measurement of physicians' work, practice costs, and the cost of malpractice insurance.

Resource-Based Relative Value Scale (RBRVS or RVS) An approach to physician reimbursement based upon the time, effort, and skill each service or procedure requires from a physician when compared with other medical services or procedures.

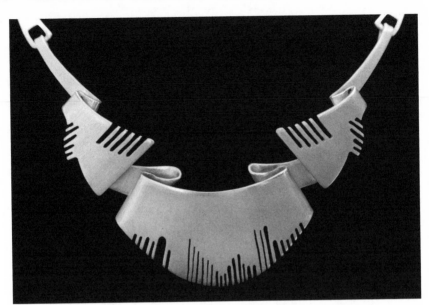

Risk Pools, Medically Uninsurable To facilitate access to healthcare services for individuals with health risks that are considered medically uninsurable, some states are creating risk pools though legislation. These are funded though a variety of mechanisms, including a premium tax on commercial insurance policies, payroll taxes, general revenues, or a combination of these approaches. Premiums for policies are usually 150 percent or more of the generally available insurance premium to avoid competing with the for-profit insurance market. Alaska has such a program.

Secondary Care Services provided by medical specialists, such as cardiologists, urologists and dermatologists, who generally do not have first contact with patients.

Self-Funding Often confused with self-insurance, a self-funded healthcare plan is funded entirely by the employer. A self-funded plan may be self-administered, or the employer may contract with an outside administrator for an administrative services only arrangement. Self-funded plans obtain stop-loss insurance to cover catastrophic illnesses.

Self-Insurance The practice of an employer or organization assuming complete responsibility for healthcare losses of its employees. This usually includes setting up a fund against which claim payments are drawn, and claims processing is often handled through an administrative service contract with an independent organization.

Self-Insured Employers who assume direct responsibility or risk for paying for employees' health care without purchasing health insurance. They usually contract with an outside firm to handle claims payment and/or utilization review.

Single-Payer System A system in which everyone is covered under a publicly run health insurance program which the government or some other single entity serves as the sole source of payment for a broad range of healthcare services.

Social Security Administration The administrative branch of the federal government established in 1935 to provide old age and survivor benefits.

Socialism Any of various theories or systems of ownership and operation of the means of production and distribution by society or the community rather than by private individuals, with all members of society or the community sharing in the work and the products. (First meaning from Webster's Dictionary). Frequently misused to describe any government program. *See also:* **Capitalism**

Socialized Medicine A system of health care wherein a government owns hospitals and pays medical providers directly, as contrasted with a capitalistic medical system wherein all hospitals are privately owned and healthcare providers operate on a fee-for-service or capitation basis, either for profit or as nonprofits. The United Kingdom has a system of socialized medicine, Canada has a capitalistic system, and the United States has a hybrid system that is mostly capitalistic.

Sole Community Hospital (SCH) A hospital which (1) is more than fifty miles from any similar hospital, (2) or is the exclusive provider of services to at least 75 percent of its service area populations or (3) has been designated as an SCH under previous rules. The Medicare DRG program makes special optional payment provisions for SCHs, most of which are rural, including providing that their rates are set permanently so that 75 percent of their payment is hospital-specific and only 25 percent is based on regional DRG rates. Fairbanks Memorial Hospital is an example.

Standard DRG Payment (Base Payment Rate) The payment per unit DRG to hospitals for Medicare services. In 2005, it was $4,570.

Super Bill A bill that lists specific and/or specialty medical services provided by a physician. Typically in a form required by Medicare or medical insurers. *See also*: **Actual Bill** and **Charge Ticket**.

Supplemental Medical Benefits Health care reform plans normally allow the acceptance of supplemental benefits, which are normally not covered by a standard benefit package. These include services not usually medically necessary such as organ transplant, or enhanced psychiatric services. Consumers would have to pay an additional premium for these benefits

Supplemental Medical Insurance Private health insurance, also called Medigap, designed to supplement Medicare benefits by covering certain healthcare costs that are not paid for by the Medicare program.

Supplemental Security Income (SSI) A federal program of income support for low income, aged, blind and disabled persons established by Title XVI of the Social Security Act. Qualification for SSI often is used to establish Medicaid eligibility.

Teaching Hospital A hospital that has an accredited medical residency training program and is typically affiliated with a medical school.

Threshold The technical term for an amount set by CMS each year that enters into the calculation of outlier payments to hospitals. (In 2003, the per patient threshold amount was $33,560.)

Traditional Health Insurance Basic health insurance that allows the policy holder to see any doctor and specialist he chooses without obtaining prior approval except perhaps for checking into a hospital for non-emergency care. Policies typically require an annual deductible and also a co-payment on all services, and the insurance company then pays the remainder of the cost of services in amounts that the company determines are reasonable.

TRICARE A health insurance system operated by the U.S. Department of Defense to serve active duty military personnel, families and military retirees. The system is separate from the Veterans Administration healthcare system. The name evidently drives from the system providing three options to beneficiaries: TRICARE standard allowing the use of any civilian healthcare provider; TRICARE Extra involving preferred provider organizations (PPOs); and TRICARE Prime which is an health maintenance organization (HMO) plan. In certain areas of the country, another option, US Family Health Plan, makes use of nonprofit providers. TRICARE contracts with several large health insurance companies to provide claims processing, customer service and other administrative functions.

U.S. Department of Health and Human Services (HHS) The federal department that regulates and administers health and human service programs in the United States. It was created in 1953 and was known as the Department of Health, Education, and Welfare until 1980 when the U.S. Department of Education was created as a separate department. The Secretary of HHS advises the president on the health, welfare, and income security plans, policies, and programs of the federal government.

Unbundling Separating a service into its individual components and billing for each component separately. Also refers to a trend in insurance benefits contracting where the purchaser unbundles or contracts separately for specific services.

Uncompensated Care The charges for services rendered by providers which are not paid for by the recipient and for which there is usually no third-party coverage. Uncompensated care is usually either charity care or bad debt.

Underinsured People with public or private insurance policies that do not cover all necessary medical services, resulting in out-of-pocket expenses that exceed their ability to pay.

Uniform National Conversion Factor (UNCF) The dollar amount (currently approximately $38) determined by congressional mandate that fixes the payment for each Current Procedural Terminology (CPT) code procedure after adjustments for geographical differences in physician pay, practice expenses, and malpractice insurance costs. *See also:* **Relative Value units (RVUs)** and **Geographic Practice Cost Indices, or Geographic Factors (GPCI).**

Uninsured Population The estimated 47 million Americans who do not have health insurance. A recent Commonwealth Fund study found that 41 percent of moderate- to middle-income adults did not have health insurance during at least a part of 2005, up from 21 percent in 2001.

Upcoding Practice of changing codes for service to higher codes for the purpose of increasing provider income—the opposite of downcoding by payers for the purpose of decreasing payments.

Veterans Administration (VA) A federal agency responsible for veterans including VA hospitals and veterans' benefits. Veterans Administration is an organizational element of the US Department of Veterans Affairs.

Workers Compensation A statutory state-operated system providing compensation to workers for medical care and lost time related to on-the-job injuries. Most employers are required to subscribe, and in most states the insurance is provided by for-profit private insurance companies.

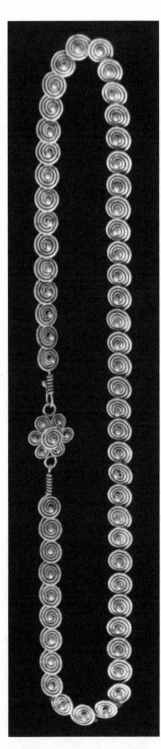

Index

Note: terms or page numbers in the Glossary are set in bold type; page numbers for terms in footnotes are indicated by 'f' after the page number.